Advanced Techniques in
PHYSIOTHERAPY AND
OCCUPATIONAL THERAPY

AF067654

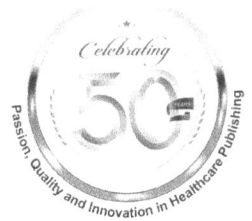

Advanced Techniques in PHYSIOTHERAPY AND OCCUPATIONAL THERAPY

Krishna N Sharma PhD MPT (Neuro) COMT (France)
Vice-Chancellor
Victoria University
Kampala, Uganda
Former Dean
St. Louis University
Bamenda, Cameroon

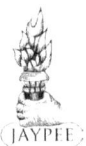

JAYPEE BROTHERS MEDICAL PUBLISHERS
The Health Sciences Publisher
New Delhi | London | Panama

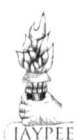 **Jaypee Brothers Medical Publishers (P) Ltd**

Headquarters
Jaypee Brothers Medical Publishers (P) Ltd
4838/24, Ansari Road, Daryaganj
New Delhi 110 002, India
Phone: +91-11-43574357
Fax: +91-11-43574314
Email: jaypee@jaypeebrothers.com

Overseas Offices

J.P. Medical Ltd
83 Victoria Street, London
SW1H 0HW (UK)
Phone: +44 20 3170 8910
Fax: +44 (0)20 3008 6180
Email: info@jpmedpub.com

Jaypee-Highlights Medical Publishers Inc
City of Knowledge, Bld. 235, 2nd Floor
Clayton, Panama City, Panama
Phone: +1 507-301-0496
Fax: +1 507-301-0499
Email: cservice@jphmedical.com

Jaypee Brothers Medical Publishers (P) Ltd
Bhotahity, Kathmandu, Nepal
Phone: +977-9741283608
Email: kathmandu@jaypeebrothers.com

Website: www.jaypeebrothers.com
Website: www.jaypeedigital.com

© 2019, Jaypee Brothers Medical Publishers

The views and opinions expressed in this book are solely those of the original contributor(s)/author(s) and do not necessarily represent those of editor(s) of the book.

All rights reserved. No part of this publication may be reproduced, stored or transmitted in any form or by any means, electronic, mechanical, photocopying, recording or otherwise, without the prior permission in writing of the publishers.

All brand names and product names used in this book are trade names, service marks, trademarks or registered trademarks of their respective owners. The publisher is not associated with any product or vendor mentioned in this book.

Medical knowledge and practice change constantly. This book is designed to provide accurate, authoritative information about the subject matter in question. However, readers are advised to check the most current information available on procedures included and check information from the manufacturer of each product to be administered, to verify the recommended dose, formula, method and duration of administration, adverse effects and contraindications. It is the responsibility of the practitioner to take all appropriate safety precautions. Neither the publisher nor the author(s)/editor(s) assume any liability for any injury and/or damage to persons or property arising from or related to use of material in this book.

This book is sold on the understanding that the publisher is not engaged in providing professional medical services. If such advice or services are required, the services of a competent medical professional should be sought.

Every effort has been made where necessary to contact holders of copyright to obtain permission to reproduce copyright material. If any have been inadvertently overlooked, the publisher will be pleased to make the necessary arrangements at the first opportunity. The **CD/DVD-ROM** (if any) provided in the sealed envelope with this book is complimentary and free of cost. **Not meant for sale.**

Inquiries for bulk sales may be solicited at: jaypee@jaypeebrothers.com

Advanced Techniques in Physiotherapy and Occupational Therapy

First Edition: **2019**
ISBN: 978-93-88958-50-9
Printed at

Contributors

A Sridhar
Professor
JDT Islam College of Physiotherapy
Kozhikode, Kerala, India

Ajay Yadav
Consultant Physiotherapist
Edmonton, Alberta, Canada
Former Associate Professor
Doon PG College
Dehradun, Uttarakhand, India

Amit M Patel
Vice-Principal
College of Physiotherapy
Ahmedabad, Gujarat, India

B Arun
Professor
KG College of Physiotherapy
Coimbatore, Tamil Nadu, India
Former Lecturer
MAHSA University
Kuala Lumpur, Malaysia

Dharam P Pandey
Director and Head
Center for Advance Physiotherapy
Sports and Neurorehabilitation
BLK Super Speciality Hospital
New Delhi, India

Divya Midha
Senior Research Fellow
Punjabi University
Patiala, Punjab, India

Harshita Yadav
PhD Scholar
Punjabi University
Patiala, Punjab, India

Kedar K Mate
PhD Candidate
McGill University
Montréal, Canada

Krishna N Sharma
Vice-Chancellor
Victoria University
Kampala, Uganda
Former Dean
St. Louis University
Bamenda, Cameroon

Kuki Bordoloi
Director (Academic)
Virtued Academy International
Mau, Uttar Pradesh, India
Former Vice-Principal
Jeevan Jyoti Institute of Medical Sciences
Allahabad, Uttar Pradesh, India

Manisha Uttam
PhD Scholar
Punjabi University
Patiala, Punjab, India

Mohamed Kassim Abdul Wahab
MSK and Sports Physiotherapist
CORE Physiotherapy
Bandar Seri Begawan, Brunei

Piyush Jain
Director
G-Xtreme International Academy
New Delhi, India

Sudeep Kale
President
Maharashtra State OT PT Council
Mumbai, Maharashtra, India

Associate Professor
Terna Physiotherapy College
Navi Mumbai, Maharashtra, India

Tanvi Patole
Physiotherapist
Bhagwan Mahaveer Medical Centre
Mumbai, Maharashtra, India

Preface

This book is aimed not only at physiotherapy (PT) and occupational therapy (OT) student, but also at practitioners, for whom this book is intended as a foundation to understand the basics of different advance techniques so that they may build on that.

The book is designed after considering undergraduate and postgraduate PT/OT syllabuses of several universities. Keeping in mind, the time constrains students and professionals have the in-depth precise information in this text is kept concise and is written in simple language that makes almost each chapter a 15 minutes read. To cater for the need of easy understanding and concept building, all the chapters flow in a particular manner that is recommended by experiences professors.

In my knowledge, it is the only book which encompasses more than 30 advance orthopedic/manual therapy, neurological, vestibular and cardiopulmonary physiotherapy and occupational therapy techniques.

I am very grateful to the whole team of M/s Jaypee Brothers Medical Publishers (P) Ltd, New Delhi, India, who helped and guided me, Shri Jitendar P Vij (Group Chairman), Mr Ankit Vij (Managing Director), Mr MS Mani (Group President), Dr Madhu Choudhary (Publishing Head–Education), Ms Pooja Bhandari (Production Head), Ms Sunita Katla (Executive Assistant to Group Chairman and Publishing Manager), Ms Samina Khan (Executive Assistant to Publishing Head–Education), Mr Rajesh Sharma (Production Coordinator), Ms Seema Dogra (Cover Visualizer), Mr Laxmidhar Padhiary (Proofreader), Mr Nitin Bhardwaj (Graphic Designer), Mr Akshay Thakur (Typesetter).

At the end, I would like to thank my wife Dr Ankita Kashyap and lovely daughter Arisha Sharma, who constantly supported to make this book possible.

Krishna N Sharma

Contents

1. **Manual Therapy** — 1
   Krishna N Sharma
2. **Kaltenborn-Evjenth Orthopedic Manual Therapy** — 10
   Krishna N Sharma
3. **Mulligan Concept** — 15
   Krishna N Sharma
4. **Maitland's Mobilization** — 19
   B Arun
5. **Cyriax Mobilization Techniques** — 24
   Ajay Yadav
6. **McKenzie Method of Mechanical Diagnosis and Therapy** — 33
   Krishna N Sharma
7. **Osteopathy** — 37
   Krishna N Sharma
8. **Chiropractic** — 41
   Kuki Bordoloi
9. **Krishna's Kinetikinetic Manual Therapy®** — 47
   Krishna N Sharma
10. **Translatoric Spinal Manipulation™** — 50
    Krishna N Sharma
11. **Matos Maneuver** — 52
    Krishna N Sharma
12. **Visceral Manipulation** — 54
    Krishna N Sharma
13. **Strain Counterstrain** — 57
    Harshita Yadav
14. **Facilitated Positional Release** — 63
    Kedar K Mate

15. **Instrument Assisted Soft Tissue Mobilization** 67
    Mohamed Kassim Abdul Wahab
16. **Stretching Techniques** 75
    Krishna N Sharma
17. **Muscle Energy Technique** 79
    Krishna N Sharma
18. **Myofascial Release** 85
    Krishna N Sharma
19. **Trigger Point Release** 92
    Amit M Patel
20. **Kinesiological Taping** 104
    Piyush Jain
21. **Pilates** 116
    Tanvi Patole
22. **Rood's Approach** 119
    Divya Midha
23. **Bobath Concept/Neurodevelopmental Treatment** 132
    Krishna N Sharma
24. **Brunnstrom Movement Therapy** 136
    Krishna N Sharma
25. **Vojta Therapy** 141
    Krishna N Sharma
26. **Motor Relearning Program** 145
    Krishna N Sharma
27. **Proprioceptive Neuromuscular Facilitation** 148
    Kuki Bordoloi, Manisha Uttam, Harshita Yadav
28. **Neurokinetic Therapy**™ 173
    Krishna N Sharma
29. **Sensory Integration Therapy** 174
    A Sridhar
30. **Graded Motor Imagery** 180
    Manisha Uttam

31. **Postural Drainage**	**186**
Sudeep Kale	
32. **Vestibular Rehabilitation**	**195**
Dharam P Pandey	
Index	*221*

CHAPTER 1

Manual Therapy

Krishna N Sharma

DEFINITIONS

Manual therapy is a clinical approach utilizing skilled, specific hands-on techniques, including but not limited to manipulation/mobilization to diagnose and treat soft tissues and joint structures for the purpose of modulating pain; increasing range of motion (ROM); reducing or eliminating soft tissue inflammation; inducing relaxation; improving contractile and non-contractile tissue repair, extensibility, and/or stability; facilitating movement; and improving function.

HISTORY (FIG. 1.1)

- Acharya Susrutha (600 BC) in his book Susrutha Samhita explained 107 marma points in the body that can be treated with the finger pressure.
- Hippocrates (460–355 BC) explained traction and few other manual therapy techniques.

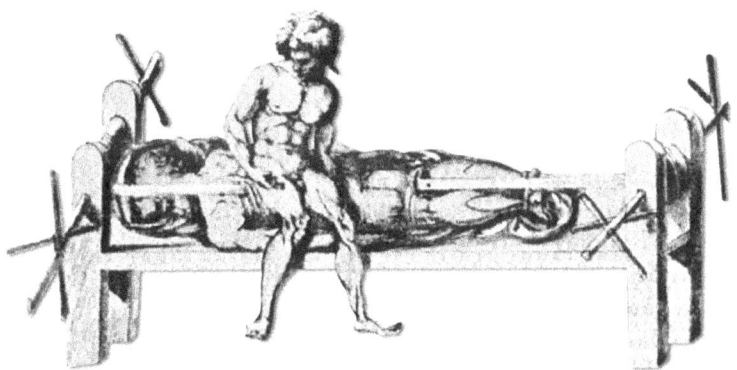

Fig. 1.1: *Hippocratic bench* or *Scamnum* invented by Hippocrates.

- Galen (131–202 AD) explained few manual therapy techniques for cervical vertebrae, as well as the upper and lower extremities.
- John Hunter (1728–1793) recommended stretching and joint movements in the cases of stiffness and adhesion.
- Bone setting flourished in Britain during the 17th and 18th centuries.
- Sir James Paget (1814–1899) suggested the medical community to learn bone setting to imitate what is good and avoid what is bad.
- Andrew Taylor Still (1828–1917) founded osteopathy in 1874 in the USA.
- Daniel David Palmer founded Chiropractic in 1895.
- Edgar and James Cyriax, and James & John Mennell taught manual therapy to the physiotherapists in beginning of the 19th century.
- Edgar Cyriax published a paper Manual Treatment of the Cervical Sympathetics in 1917.
- Walmsley coined the term Arthrokinametics in 1927.
- James Mennell wrote a book "Manual Therapy" and got published in 1951.
- James Cyriax published a book "Textbook of Orthopaedic Medicine" in 1954. His book made the term End Feel popular.
- John Mennell used the term Joint Play for the first time in his book "Joint Pain" published in 1960.
- Kaltenborn linked the arthrokinematics with the manual therapy and published his book "Extremity Joint Manipulation" in 1961.
- Stanley V Paris published "Theory and Technique of Specific Spinal Manipulation" in 1963.
- Geoffrey Maitland published his book "Vertebral Manipulation" in 1964.
- In 1966, Kaltenborn, Paris, Grieve, and Maitland held a meeting which resulted into the foundation of Federation of Orthopaedic Manual Therapy (IFOMT).
- In the late 1970s, McKenzie introduced his own concept.

TYPES OF MANUAL THERAPY
According to the Application
- Joint:
    - Mobilization

- Manipulation
- Traction, etc.
- Muscle:
  - Soft tissue manipulation
  - Muscle energy technique, etc.
- Neural structure:
  - Neural stretching.

According to the Procedures
- Thrust:
  - High velocity thrust technique/manipulation
- Non-thrust:
  - Graded oscillations
  - Stretching
  - Soft tissue manipulation
  - Myofascial release
  - Muscle energy technique, etc.

EFFECTS OF MANUAL THERAPY
- Biomechanical effects:
  - Joint displacement
  - Increase in range of motion (ROM) due to passive movements
- Muscular reflexogenic effects:
  - Muscular inhibition
  - Muscular facilitation
- Neurophysiologic effects:
  - Pain inhibition and analgesia
  - Pain gate mechanism
- Psychological effects:
  - Placebo.

TERMINOLOGY
Mobilization
Mobilization is passive joint movement applied to spinal or peripheral joint in which a rhythmic oscillatory movement within the control of patient is applied at varying speeds and amplitudes using physiologic or accessory motions to increase range of motion (ROM) or decreasing pain.

Manipulation

Manipulation is passive joint movement applied to a joint in which a sudden, forceful thrust beyond the patient's control is applied to increase range of motion (ROM).

Soft Tissue Manipulation

The soft tissue manipulation techniques involve various forms of deep massage and are used to increase the mobility of adherent or shortened connective tissues.

Muscle Energy Technique

Muscle energy techniques use the concepts of autogenic inhibition, and reciprocal inhibition to relax and then stretch the target muscle. The patient is asked to do isometric/concentric/eccentric contraction in a precisely controlled direction and intensity against a counterforce applied by the therapist.

Neural Stretching

The neural tissues are stretched and mobilized in the cases of adhesion or scar tissue around the nerve root or at the site of injury at the plexus or peripheral nerves after trauma or surgical procedures. Tension placed on the adhesions or scar tissue leads to pain or neurological symptoms.

Graded Oscillation

Graded oscillation was widely promoted by Maitland. Graded oscillation is a form of cyclic loading whereby alternative pressure, on and off, is delivered at different parts of the available range.

Stretching

Stretching is a general terms that describe any therapeutic maneuver that increases the extensibility of restricted soft tissues.

Myofascial Release

Myofascial release techniques focus on relaxing the fascia by applying direct pressure on the body and using slow and sometimes deep pressure to restore the extensibility of the fascia.

SCHOOLS OF THOUGHT
Though there are various schools of thought in manual therapy, I would like to quote few notables ones.
- **Osteopathy:**
  - The founder of osteopathic medicine was Andrew Taylor Still (1827-1917).
  - Still observed through careful study of a patient that when joints are restricted in motion due to mechanical locking or other related causes were normalized, certain disease conditions improved.
  - Dr Still made the "Rule of the Artery" which says that if we manipulate to restore blood flow, it will restore body's innate healing ability.
  - According to osteopathy:
    - The body is a unit; structure and function are reciprocally interrelated.
    - The body possesses self-regulatory mechanisms for rational therapies based on an understanding of the body unity, the self-regulatory mechanisms.
    - There is interrelation of structure and function.
- **Chiropractic:**
  - Founded in 1895 by DD Palmer (1845-1913).
  - In Chiropractic "Subluxation" of the spine is a causal factor in disease and the revelation that adjustments can restore the body's innate healing abilities.
  - "Chiropractors do not manipulate; they do not use the process of manipulating; they adjust."
  - DD Palmer applied an "adjustment" to Harvey Lillard in September 1895 to the T4 vertebra that resulted in restoration of lost hearing.
  - Palmer School of Chiropractic founded in 1897 in Davenport, Iowa.
- **Williams:**
  - Dr Paul Williams observed that the majority of patients who experienced low back pain had degenerative vertebrae secondary to degenerative disc disease.
  - He first published his exercise program in 1937 for patients with chronic low back pain.

- These exercises were developed for men under 50 and women under 40 years of age:
    - Who had exaggerated lumbar lordosis
    - Whose X-ray films showed decreased disc space between lumbar spine segments (L1-S1)
    - Whose symptoms were chronic but low grade.
- His exercises were flexion biased.
- The goals of performing Williams exercises are to reduce pain and provide lower trunk stability by actively developing the "abdominal, gluteus maximus, and hamstring muscles as well as passively stretching the hip flexors and lower back (sacrospinalis) muscles.
- Williams said: "*The exercises outlined will accomplish a proper balance between the flexor and the extensor groups of postural muscles.*"
- Conceptually, Williams felt that the goal of exercise was to reduce the lumbar lordosis or to flatten the back.
- To do this, he suggested strengthening the abdominal muscles in order to lift the pelvis from the front.
- In addition, he proposed strengthening the gluteal muscles would pull the back of the pelvis down.
- According to Williams, the combination of these two exercises would accomplish the primary goal of flattening the lumbar curve.

- **Mennell:**
    - Published his book in 1951.
    - Felt that 'joint play' is key to normal function.
    - He emphasized the importance of the small accessory movements as necessary for full movement to occur.
    - Techniques are more specific for the extremities than for the spine.
    - He was one of the first clinicians to study the intimate mechanics of joints and to adapt mobilizations to his findings.
    - He coined the term accessory motion.
- **Cyriax:**
    - Founded by James Cyriax.
    - Used selective tension techniques to identify faulty structures in the examination.
    - Emphasized the need for soft tissue massage and frequently used injection of muscle trigger points.

Manual Therapy

- Believed the disc is the primary cause of low back pain and used nonspecific spinal techniques designed to move the disc to relive nerve root pressure.
- Started to use the term cross friction.
- Also known for the term endfeel.
- He published a book "Textbook of Orthopaedic Medicine" in 1954.

- **Kaltenborn**
  - Freddy Kaltenborn is known for his research in arthrokinematics.
  - He gave different classification of joints for manual therapists.
  - His techniques incorporate the influence of muscle function and soft-tissue changes in the patient's manifestation of loss of function.
  - Kaltenborn published his book "Extremity Joint Manipulation" in 1961.

- **Maitland:**
  - Founded by Geoffrey Maitland.
  - Used primarily passive accessory movements to restore function.
  - Relies on an extensive assessment based on information from the patient's subjective examination (history) and the evaluator's objective assessment.
  - The movements are oscillations, the techniques are specific and the goals is what he terms 'reproducible signs'.
  - The Maitland concept is referred to as a 'concept' and not as a 'technique'.
  - He published his book "Vertebral Manipulation" in 1964.

- **McKenzie:**
  - Robin Anthony McKenzie noted that a subset of his patients experienced significant pain relief when the spine was extended as the part of a treatment. Often, these patients were able to return to normal daily activities.
  - Physical therapists who practiced the methods developed by McKenzie founded the McKenzie Institute in 1982.
  - This modality may be used to treat any number of back, spine, muscle, bone, or joint disorders.
  - In order to determine if the McKenzie Method® will relieve a patient's pain or improve their mobility or range of motion, the patient attempts several of the exercises designed to reduce the sensation of pain.

- If the pain moves towards the spine or is eliminated, then the patient may be an appropriate candidate for the McKenzie Method®.
- Centralization is the term practitioners of this modality use to describe this movement or elimination of pain.
- Usually, if the patient's pain and spinal-related problems do not have a mechanical origin, the McKenzie Method® may not be a useful treatment for that individual.
- McKenzie is a comprehensive approach to the spine based on sound principles and fundamentals that when understood and followed accordingly are very successful.
- The McKenzie method: Three steps to success:
    1. Assessment
    2. Treatment
    3. Prevention

- **Mulligan:**
    - Developed and founded by Brian Mulligan.
    - In 1983 Brian began teaching his techniques.
    - For extremities: MWMs (Mobilization with movement)
    - For spine: NAGs (Natural apophyseal glides) and SNAGs (Sustained natural apophyseal glides).
    - The patient is requested to perform the comparable sign (by performing a classic movement). These signs may be a loss of joint movement, pain associated with movement, or pain associated with specific functional activities.
    - A passive accessory joint mobilization is applied. This accessory glide must itself be pain free.
    - The comparable sign should now be significantly improved (i.e. increased range of motion, and a significantly decreased or better yet, absence of the original pain).
    - The previously restricted and/or painful motion or activity is repeated by the patient while the therapist continues to maintain the appropriate accessory glide.
    - Failure to improve the comparable sign would indicate that the therapist has not found the correct contact point, treatment plane, grade or direction of mobilization, spinal segment or that the technique is not indicated.

- **Krishna's Kinetikinetic Manual Therapy (KKMT):**
    - Developed by Dr Krishna N Sharma in 2015.
    - Based on 7 principles.

Manual Therapy

- Realigns and harmonizes the incongruity and altered states of body, mind, and energy by manipulating the homeostatic kinetic forces and energies.
- The KKMT protocol includes *assessment*, *mobilization*, and *prevention*. Each of these are done separately for three aspects of a human being, i.e. *body*, *mind*, and *energies*.
- Though a therapist can work on any of these three aspect, working on all of them is recommended for better outcome.

CHAPTER

2 Kaltenborn-Evjenth Orthopedic Manual Therapy

Krishna N Sharma

HISTORY

It was originally developed by *Mr Freddy M Kaltenborn* from Norway who later on collaborated with another Norwegian practitioner *Mr Olaf Evjenth* in 1958 who contributed in this school of thought by developing techniques for muscle strengthening, stretching and coordination training (Fig. 2.1).

- Mr Kaltenborn started his career as a physical educator and athletic trainer in Germany in 1945.
- He started working as a physical therapist in Norway in 1949.
- He worked as a Physical Therapist in Norway from 1950 to 1982.
- Between 1952 and 1954, he worked with Dr James Mennell and Dr James Cyriax in St. Thomas Hospital, London, England.

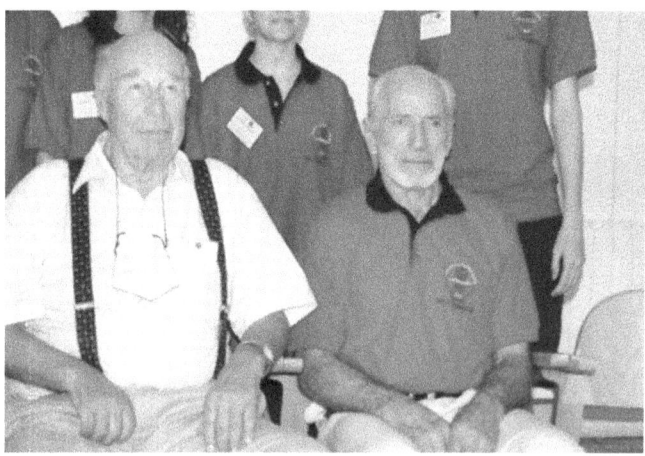

Fig. 2.1: Mr Freddy M Kaltenborn (left) and Mr Olaf Evjenth (right).

Kaltenborn-Evjenth Orthopedic Manual Therapy

- This system began in 1954 with joint testing and treatment and was known as *Manual Therapy ad Modum Kaltenborn*.
- It later became known as the *Nordic System* or Norwegian System.
- He became certified instructor if Cyriax approach in 1955.
- After this he studied at the British School of Osteopathy.
- After returning to his native country Norway, he started incorporating these learned concepts into his own system.
- In 1958, the physical therapists in Norway referred his techniques as *Manual Therapy ad Modum Kaltenborn*.
- Kaltenborn also studied chiropractic and became certified in 1958 by the Forschungs- und Arbeitsgemeinschaft für Chiropraktik (FAC) in Germany.
- In 1962 the FAC incorporated the *Kaltenborn Method* into their approach and changed the name of their professional practice from "Chiropraktik" to "Chirotherapy."
- In 1962 he studied at the London College of Osteopathy in London, England.
- He published his first book on manual therapy *Frigjøring av Ryggraden* in Norwegian language in 1964.
- This book was translated in English by Robin McKenzie and was published as *Mobilization of the Spine*, 1970.
- In 1971, he became certified osteopathic instructor by Dr Alan Stoddard.
- He published his second book *Manual Therapy for the Extremity Joints* in 1974.
- He presented his *OMT Kaltenborn-Evjenth Concept* in 1973 when he with Cyriax, Hinsen, and Stoddard founded *International Seminar of Orthopaedic Manipulative Therapy (ISOMT)*.
- Between 1977 and 1984 he served as a professor at the Michigan State University, College of Osteopathic Medicine, USA.

KALTENBORN-EVJENTH OMT PROTOCOL

This concept has its standard protocol and the techniques are just a part of this protocol. This concept follows the following protocol taken from the 4th edition of his book *Manual Mobilization of Joints—The Kaltenborn Method of Joint Examination and Treatment, Volume II—The Spine*.

Physical Diagnosis (Biomechanical and Functional Assessment)

A. **Screening Examination:** A short exam to quickly identify the region with problem.
B. **Detailed Examination**
   1. **History:** Narrow diagnostic possibilities; develop early hypotheses to be confirmed by further examination; determine whether or not symptoms are musculoskeletal and treatable with OMT (includes present episode, past medical history, related personal history, family history, review of systems).
   2. **Inspection:** Further focus the examination (includes posture, shape, skin, assistive devices).
   3. **Tests of function:**
      a. **Active and passive movements:** Identify location, type, and severity of dysfunction (includes standard-anatomical-uniaxial movements and combined-functional-multiaxial movements).
      b. **Translatoric joint play movements:** Further differentiate articular from nonarticular lesions; identify directions of joint restrictions (includes traction, compression, gliding).
      c. **Resisted movements:** Test neuromuscular integrity and status of associated joints, nerves and vascular supply.
      d. **Passive soft tissue movements:** Differentiate joint from soft tissue dysfunction and the type of soft tissue involvement (includes physiological movements, accessory movements).
      e. **Additional tests** (includes coordination, speed, endurance, functional capacity assessment).
   4. **Palpation** (includes tissue characteristics, structures).
   5. **Neurologic and vascular examination.**
C. Medical diagnostic studies (includes diagnostic imaging, laboratory tests, electrodiagnostic tests, punctures).
D. Diagnosis and trial treatment.

Treatment

To Relieve Symptoms (Most Often Pain)
1. **Immobilization**
   - General—bed rest
   - Specific—corsets, splinting, casting, taping
2. **Thermo-Hydro-Electro (T-H-E) therapy**
3. **Pain relief joint mobilization** (Grade /-1/ Slack Zone in the actual resting position)
   - Intermittent manual traction
   - Vibrations, oscillations.
4. **Special procedures** (Includes acupuncture, acupressure, soft tissue mobilization).

To Increase Mobility
1. **Soft tissue mobilization**
   a. **Passive soft tissue mobilization**
      - Classical, functional, and friction massage.
   b. **Active-facilitated soft tissue mobilization**
      - Contract-relax, reciprocal inhibition, muscle stretching.
2. **Joint mobilization**
   a. **Relaxation joint mobilization (Grade I–II)**
      - Three-dimensional, pre-positioned mobilizations.
   b. **Stretch joint mobilization (Grade III)**
      - Manual mobilization in the joint (actual) resting position
      - Manual mobilization at the point of restriction.
   c. **Manipulation**
      - High velocity, short amplitude, linear thrust movement.
3. **Neural tissue mobilization:** To increase mobility of dura mater, nerve roots, and peripheral nerves.
4. **Specialized exercise:** To increase or maintain soft tissue length and mobility and joint mobility.

To Limit Movement
1. **Supportive devices.**
2. **Specialized exercise.**
3. **Treatments to increase movement in adjacent joints.**

To Inform, Instruct, and Train

Exercises and education to improve function, compensate for injuries, and prevent reinjury. Instruction in relevant ergonomics and self-care techniques, e.g. medical training therapy, automobilization, autostabilization, autostretching, back school, activities of daily living, etc.

Research

Clinical trials to determine the efficacy of both single and combined treatment methods. An evidence-based approach to every aspect of evaluation and treatment is an essential precursor to orthopedic manual therapy (OMT) research.

CHAPTER 3

Mulligan Concept

Krishna N Sharma

HISTORY

Mulligan concept (sometimes referred as Mulligan techniques) was introduces by Brian R Mulligan, a physiotherapist qualified in 1954. He was introduced to manual therapy by Stanley Paris in the early 1960s. He began teaching his techniques in 1983 (Fig. 3.1).

CONCEPTS

Concept of Positional Fault

Injuries might result in a minor "positional fault" to a joint that causes restrictions in physiological movement due to tracking problems. This altered joint position/tracking during movement provokes symptoms of pain, stiffness or weakness in the patient. These restrictions can be treated by solving the 'positional faults'.

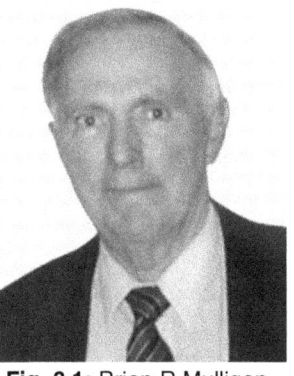

Fig. 3.1: Brian R Mulligan.

Concept of Mobilization with Movement

It is the concurrent application of sustained accessory mobilization applied by a therapist and an active physiological movement to end range applied by the patient. Passive end-of-range overpressure, or stretching, is then delivered without pain as a barrier.

PRINCIPLES OF TREATMENT

- The patient is requested to perform the comparable sign (by performing a classic movement). These signs may be a loss of joint movement, pain associated with movement, or pain associated with specific functional activities.

- A pain free passive joint glide is applied.
- The comparable sign should now be significantly improved (i.e. increased range of motion, and a significantly decreased or better yet, absence of the original pain).
- The patient must show **PILL** response (**P**—Pain free, **I**—Instant result, **LL**—Long Lasting). Absence of PILL response indicates that the either the therapist has not found the correct contact point, treatment plane, grade or direction of mobilization, spinal segment; or the technique is contraindicated.
- The previously restricted and/or painful motion or activity is repeated by the patient while the therapist continues to maintain the appropriate accessory glide.

CROCKS Principle

C—**C**ontraindications (No PILL response is a contraindication)
R—**R**epetitions (only three repetitions on the day one)
O—**O**ver pressure at the end range
C—**C**ommunications
K—**K**nowledge of treatment planes and pathologies
S—**S**ustain the mobilization throughout the movement.

TECHNIQUES

For Spine

Natural Apophyseal Glides

- *Natural apophyseal glides (NAGs):* These are used for cervical and upper thoracic spine. It consists of mid-range to end-range oscillatory mobilizations and it can be applied to the facet joints between C2 and D3/T3. In this, the superior facet glides up the inferior. The glide is applied anterosuperiorly along the treatment planes.
- *Reverse NAGs:* It is used when NAGs is unsuccessful. In this technique, the inferior facet glides up on the superior.
- *Sustained natural apophyseal glides (SNAGs)*:
  - It is most effective when the symptoms are provoked by movements. The therapist glides the specific facet while the patient performs the symptomatic movement. This must result in full range pain free movement.

Mulligan Concept

- ♦ Cervical flexion SNAG
- ♦ Cervical extension SNAG
- ♦ Cervical rotation SNAG
- – Self-SNAGs
- – *Headache SNAGs:* It is useful in the patients with cervicogenic headache. It restores the loss of C1 and C2 rotations.
    - ♦ Headache SNAGs
    - ♦ Reverse headache SNAGs
    - ♦ Self-headache SNAGs
- *Spinal mobilization with arm movements (SMWAMs):*
    - – *SMWAMs:* It is useful when the pain radiates to the upper extremity. In this techniques, arm movements are combined with sustained cervical spinal mobilization.
    - – Self-SMWAMs
- *Spinal mobilization with leg movements (SMWLMs):* It is useful when the pain radiates to the lower extremity. In this techniques, leg movements are combined with sustained lumbar spinal mobilization.
- *Traction techniques*
    - – *Fist tractions:* This is used when the patient experiences pain in mid-to-end range neck flexion.
    - – *Upper cervical traction:* It is upper cervical traction with slight extension.
    - – *Belt traction techniques:* Mulligan belt is used to apply traction from the mid-thoracic to lumbar spines.
    - – Self-traction
- *Leg raise techniques*
    - – Bent leg raise technique (BLR)
    - – Two leg rotation technique
    - – Straight leg raise with traction
    - – Straight leg raise with compression
- *Taping*

For Extremities

- *Mobilization with movements (MWMs)*
    - – MWMs: *It is useful in the peripheral joints. In this techniques, the joint is glided/rotated/or distracted with active movement of the same joint.*

- MWMs with glide
- MWMs with rotation
- MWMs with distraction
  - *Self MWMs:* These can be performed by the patients themselves.
- *Pain release phenomenon (PRP)*
  - Compression treatments
    - Compression technique
    - Squeeze technique
- *Taping.*

CHAPTER

5 Maitland's Mobilization

B Arun

The Maitland concept (Techniques) of manipulative physiotherapy emphasizes a specific way of thinking, continuous evaluation and assessment and the art of manipulative physiotherapy and a total commitment to the patient (Fig. 4.1).
—*International Maitland Teachers Association, 2013*

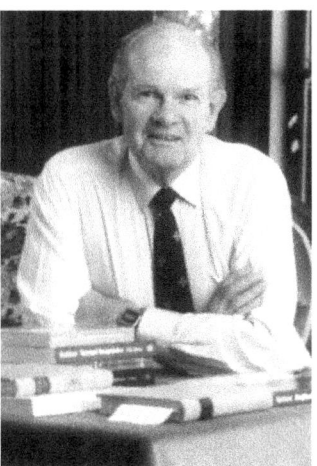

Fig. 4.1: Geoffrey Maitland.

MOBILIZATION
Mobilizations are the passive movements executed by physiotherapist at a slow speed so that patient can stop or control the movements.

MANIPULATIONS
Manipulations are the sudden movements executed with a high velocity (speed), short amplitude motions so that patient cannot prevent the movements.

INDICATIONS
- Pain
- Stiffness
- Hypomobility
- Muscle spasm
- Reduce functionally mobility.

CONTRAINDICATIONS
- Inflammatory arthritis (RA, AKS)
- Osteoporosis
- Vertebral artery problems (VBI)
- Malignancy
- Spondylolisthesis
- Vertebral stenosis
- Sever nerve root compression
- Recent fractures
- Undiagnosed pain/idiopathic pain
- Pregnancy
- Unstable spine
- Psychological pain
- Long-term use of steroids.

CAUSES FOR COMPLICATIONS
- Therapist-related complications
  - Poor diagnosis
  - Poor skills in manipulation
  - No interpersonal consultations
- Patient-related complications
  - Patient involved in any litigations
  - Patient with psychological intolerance of pain
  - Dependence on manipulation (Patient comfortable with mobilization)
  - Uncomplicated sciatica or any radiating pain or any sensory loss.

JOINT POSITIONS IN MOBILIZATION TECHNIQUES
- Joint play
  - Each joint in the body has positioned to make maximum amount of motion.
  - Joint should be positioned in a relaxed position.
- Resting position:
  - This is the position in which the joint capsule and ligaments are relaxed. This position help in evaluation of the joint.
  - This position is selected for the management of hypo-mobile joint.

- Placing the joint in resting position allows the joint to assumes a loose pack position.
- Closed pack position:
  - This is the position where there is a maximal contact of articular surface of bones with capsule and ligaments are tense or tight.
  - This is the position where there is no movement is seen.

TREATMENT PLANES

Movements are directed as per treatment planes. Treatment plane is an imaginary line parellel to joint surface. The direction of motion is either parallel or perpendicular to the treatment planes. Usually joint tractions are perpendicular to the treatment plane and the joint glides are parallel to the treatment planes (Fig. 4.2).

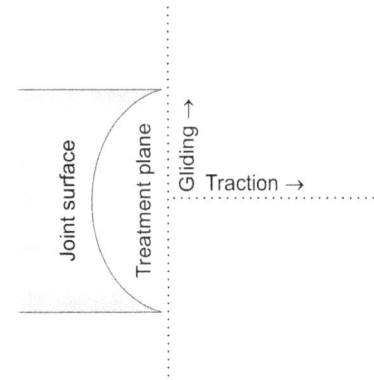

Fig. 4.2: Treatment plane.

GRADES OF MOBILIZATION

Grading of the mobilization is based on the amplitude of movement on the available range of motion and the amount of force applied to the joint.
- Grade I: Small amplitude of rhythmic oscillating movements at the starting range of movement.
- Grade II: Large amplitude rhythmic oscillating movement within the midrange of movement.
- Grade III: Large amplitude rhythmic oscillating movement up to point of limitation (PL) in range of movement.
- Grade IV: Small amplitude rhythmic oscillating movement at very **end** range of movement.
- Grade V (thrust technique): Manipulation, small amplitude, quick thrust at end of range accompanied by popping sound (manipulation).
- Grades I and II for reducing pain.
- Grades III and IV for improving the range of motion.

CONCAVE–CONVEX RULES

Concave convex rule is based on the joint morphology:
- Rule I: When the concave articular structure is moving on the convex articular structure, then the rolling, gliding and bone movement occurs in the same directions, e.g. knee joint, elbow joint (Fig. 4.3).
- Rule II: When the convex articular structure is moving on the concave articular structure, then the rolling, and bone movement occurs in the same directions whereas gliding occurs in opposite directions, e.g. shoulder joint, hip joint (Fig. 4.4).

EFFECT OF MOBILIZATION

- **Stiffness is reduced by the principle of:**
  - Mobilization showed that it helps in breakdown of muscle shortening and reduce the fibroblastic proliferations inside the joints.

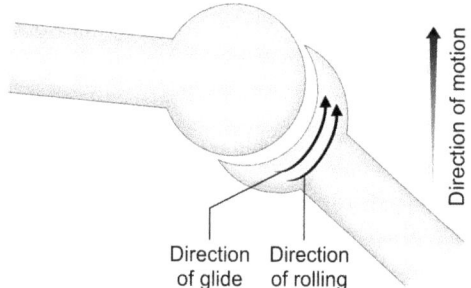

Fig. 4.3: Concave surface moving on convex surface.

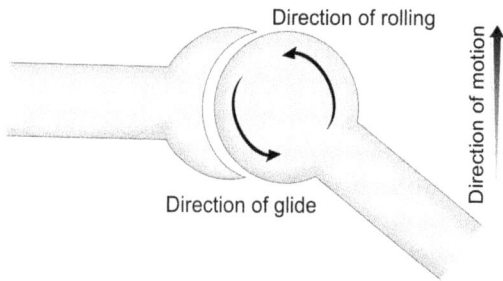

Fig. 4.4: Convex surface moving on concave surface.

- Forceful passive movements have shown to rupture of intra-articular adhesion that forms during immobilization.
- **Pain reduction occurs as a result of:**
  - During oscillatory glides, faster impulses overwhelm the slower impulses. It helps in closing of gate at spinal level. Release of endorphins from central nervous system (CNS).

CHAPTER 5

Cyriax Mobilization Techniques

Ajay Yadav

HISTORY

Dr James H Cyriax, MD, MRCP (1904–1985), an orthopedic surgeon in London, was the first to approach the study of soft tissue injuries in a thorough and systemic way. Cyriax dedicated his professional life to improve not only his own skills but also those of "indifferent" physical therapists and medical physicians. His greatest gift to both professions is found in his classic book Textbook of Orthopedics Medicine, Volume I, originally published in 1954. In this book he laid out the foundation of a method of logical, clinically reasoned, differential diagnosis, which he called "selective tissue tension testing (Fig. 5.1)."

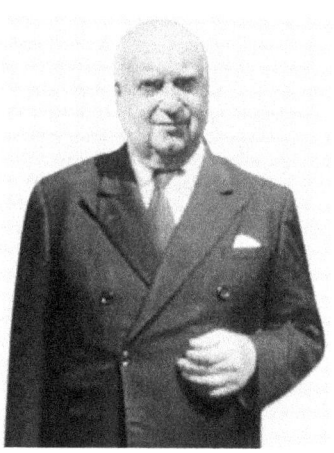

Fig. 5.1: Dr James H Cyriax.

PRINCIPLES

- All pain arises from a lesion.
- All treatment must reach the affected site.
- All treatment must exert a beneficial effect on the affected site.

Core Concept

1. **A good understanding of the phenomenon "referred pain":** The chief obstacle to correct diagnosis in painful conditions is the fact that the symptom is often felt at a distance from its source. The diagnosis will often turn on the assessment of the site and nature

of the pain and the manner in which it is projected and elicited. In the Cyriax concept, referred pain obeys certain rules. The inadequacy in the sensory cortex is structural and therefore can easily be accommodated. To a certain degree, referred pain can be compared with the refraction of light when it falls on a water surface. The observer does not see objects under the water surface at their exact localization. However, since the error of perception is structural and obeys particular physical rules and laws, it is easy to correct what is seen (provided the observer knows the correction formula) and so locate the object accurately.

2. **Examination by selective tissue tension:** Cyriax had to begin somewhere, so he started with the simple assumption that if a damaged tissue was pulled it would hurt, tension on the structure would give rise to pain, wherever that pain might be felt. If each structure acting on or around a joint could be put under tension independently and in turn, then the structure at fault could be identified. This simple postulate turned out to be extremely effective. He worked out that some tissues (the contractile tissues, the muscles with their associated tendons, nerve and bony insertion) could be made to apply tension to themselves by a simple strong isometric contraction. The inert structures (joint capsule, ligaments, bursae) would not have been moved during this contraction, but could, by contrast, be put under tension by being stretched passively. A logical system of examination was developing, and would become known as "Examination by Selective Tissue Tension". Accurate clinical observation next showed him that when inflammation of a joint was present (synovitis or capsulitis), not only would passive stretching of the capsule be painful but limitation of range was always in a specific pattern; this pattern was always similar for that particular joint, although each joint has a different and instantly recognizable capsular pattern.

Cyriax had three principles for examination by selective tissue tension:
1. Isometric contractions test the function of the contractile tissues.
2. Passive movements test the function of the inert structures.
3. Capsular patterns differentiate between joint conditions and other inert structure lesions.

Cyriax Divide Tissues into Contractile and Non-contractile

Contractile Structure

It includes muscles and its attachment. From these structures pain may be elicited by active contraction as well as passive stretching in opposite directions.

Non-contractile

These tissues posses no inherent capacity to contract and relax. The agency of movement lies outside themselves. Extreme range of active movements will stretch the structures causing pain. He emphasized testing the muscle to elicit maximum strength while the joint in its most relaxed, neutral position to reduce joint compression. Testing a muscle in its neutral position eliminates the pain of impingement and instability.

Capsular Pattern

A distinctive feature of the Cyriax method is the capsular pattern. This *capsular pattern* denotes inflammation of the capsule such as in an inflammatory or traumatic arthritis, a fracture or a cancer which extends close to or into that joint. It is associated with a specific pattern of limitation with the various passive movements at the joint. Each joint has its own distinctive capsular pattern. A *non-capsular* pattern implies that the capsule is not involved and that intra- or extra-articular tissue is inflamed or injured and the source of pain.

TREATMENT

Treatment depends largely on the existing type of disorder and can be categorized as: Traumatic, inflammatory, degenerative, internal derangement, functional disorders, psychogenic pain.

The types of treatment options are:
- *Deep friction:* It is useful technique in treating traumatic and overuses soft tissue lesions.
- *Active movements and proprioceptive training:* These are used in the treatment of functional disorders and instability. They are very useful in avoiding the formation of abnormal intra-lesional adhesion formation in minor tears.
- *Passive movements:* These are used to stretch capsular adhesions to improve the function of ligaments and tendons. It is often used

Cyriax Mobilization Techniques

in combination with deep transverse massage for the treatment of traumatic injuries.
- *Manipulation techniques:* These are used to reduce small cartilaginous displaced fragments both in the spine and in peripheral joints (loose bodies).
- *Injection and infiltration techniques:* These are used to reduce traumatic or rheumatoid inflammation. They are mostly required in arthritis, bursitis, ligamentous and tendinous lesions and in neurocompression syndromes.

DEEP FRICTION

Effects of Deep Friction Massage
- Increased blood supply relieves pain. Deep friction results in more lasting hyperemia and appears to be in this way that friction itself is painful. Deep friction massage given to a lesion gives temporary analgesia.
- By moving the painful structure to and fro, it can be freed from adhesion. Present and process of formation of adhesions. It is applied along the length of fibers. Transverse friction massage does not disrupt the fibers joining the joint like ligaments. It is moved in the limitation of normal behavior but not stretched.
- It increases tissue perfusion at damaged area and stimulates the mechanoreceptor cells.

Indications
Prevention of adhesion formation, pain relief, promotes healing for muscle tears, for treating ankle and knee sprains, for capsules of trapezium, 1st metacarpal joints, temporomandibular joint (TMJ) and cervical facet joint, defines exact location of lesion.

Contraindications
Ulcer, psoriasis, blisters, hematoma, bacterial and rheumatoid disorders, disorder of nerve structures.

Technique
Cyriax's description of friction massage offered two forms of treatment. The first in the **longitudinal** in which the application of force runs parallel to fibers of the soft tissue structures. The second

is **transverse** friction massage in which the force is applied perpendicular to the fibers, an attempt to separate each fiber, mechanically assisting in alignment of newly-formed collagen during healing.

While treating patient the therapeutic movement should be applied to the exact site of the lesion, to find the point that reproduces the patient's pain.

Friction should be applied with sufficient sweep to reach all the affected tissue and enough to produce movement between the individual connective tissue fibers of the affected structure.

Attention must be paid to different elements such as the position of the patient and of the therapist's hand.

Position of the Patient

The patient's position must be comfortable and the lesion must be within finger's reach. Full relaxation is necessary for a muscle belly in order not only to treat its surface but also to access a deeply seated lesion. Tendons with a sheath must be kept taut.

Position of the Therapist and the Hands

The position of the patient should be comfortable, therapist should avoid flexed positions. Movement is generated in the shoulder and conducted via elbow and forearm to the digits. The majority of friction techniques are performed in two phases: *an active movement*, usually as a result of flexor muscular activity and a *passive movement*, when the arm and hand are returned to the starting position. At the end of the passive phase there should also be a moment of rest during which the therapist fully relaxes the muscles.
Three main techniques can be distinguished.

To-and-fro Movements

These are used in the treatment of dense, round or flat collagenous bundles (tendons or ligaments) and in the treatment of tenosynovitis. The active phase is a sweep with the tip of one or two digits across the tendinous structure. During the passive relaxation phase the finger is returned to the starting position, without losing contact between finger and skin. Movement is with the arm; friction is given by use of the pulpy part of the finger. In large lesions, as in peroneal tendinitis, two or three adjacent fingers are used together. In deep-seated lesions as in tendinitis of the long head of biceps in the bicipital groove or at its insertion on the radius or in infraspinatus tendinitis, the thumb performs friction.

Pronation–supination

This technique is often used where the lesion is difficult to reach: the anterior aspect of the Achilles tendon, popliteus tendon and the dorsal interossei of the metacarpals. Massage is performed with the pulpy part of the third finger (long finger), reinforced by the index finger. The long finger is used because its long axis is the prolongation of the axis of pronation-supination rotation of the forearm.

The active phase is usually on supination. No counterpressure is given. Caution is taken not to move the finger on the skin but rather to move the skin and the fingertip as a whole. The passive phase is the pronation movement that brings the frictioning finger back to the starting position without losing contact with the skin.

Pinch Grip

This is the normal technique for a muscle belly. The pinch is between the thumb and the other fingers. The muscle is fully relaxed. The fingers are placed at one side of the affected area and the thumb at the opposite side. By drawing the fingers upwards over the affected area, the therapist feels the muscle fibers escape from the grip until only skin and subcutaneous tissue remain.

During the passive phase the fingers are slightly relaxed and moved downwards into the previous deep position where the same sometimes the same technique is used in tendinous lesions, for example, at the sides of the Achilles tendon.

ACTIVE MOVEMENTS

Muscles

- ***Active exercises:*** They are used to prevent adhesions forming within or about a muscle.
- ***Assisted exercises:*** Active exercises alone are ineffective but active movements in required direction is assisted by physiotherapist.
- ***Resisted exercises:*** Its purpose is to strengthening of muscle. Resistance is applied by physiotherapist by the help of pulleys and springs or by patient own limb weight.
- ***Active movements under local anesthesia:*** In treatment of muscular injury the unrestricted movement that local anesthesia secures most high value.

- ***Exercises resisted within free range:*** Useful for muscle strengthening. The technique is valuable after operations on joints especially meniscectomy at knee.

Joints

- ***Active exercises:*** They are used to retain mobility of muscle and to increase range. The main use is to keep structure normal.
- ***Passive then active movements:*** They are used to increase the range of movement in every possible direction.
- ***Static contraction and exercises to resisted that no movement occurs*:** Used to improve desirable range of joint. The increased strength of muscles diminishes articular movement, thus relieving fibrous structures from stress.
- ***Active exercise with passive effect:*** Active movements that causes passive stretching.

MANIPULATION

James Cyriax became an Honorary member and the first fellow of the British Association of Manipulative Medicine in 1975. Cyriax visualized the existence of two types of disc lesion; the annular cartilaginous fragment that he felt was the manipulative lesion; and the nucleus pulposus herniation or soft disc prolapsed, which is unlikely to be reduced by manipulation responding, however, to traction or epidural injection. Cyriax considered that intra-articular derangements occurred at the peripheral joints when they were due to loose bodies or meniscus detachments, and also at spinal joint owing to annular detachments. The correct treatment was manipulation. Usually this was a combination manual traction, a passive movement and the over-pressure. Before any manipulation is done an exact diagnosis must be made. The decision to manipulate is followed by choice of the correct maneuver. The patient is put in a comfortable position and the manipulator adopts a stable stance.

Appropriate Technique

Manipulative techniques contain important safeguards against possible accidents.

Once a manipulation has started, the operator must always concentrate on the type of *tissue resistance* (end-feel) *while taking up the slack* just before the final thrust is given. If the end-feel is abnormal, he must stop immediately and must not manipulate. To push through muscle spasm protecting a joint should never be attempted. To prevent compression of the spinal cord all manipulations must be performed under *traction*.

The major aim of manipulation should always be to gain maximal benefit with the use of minimal force. Therefore, it is good sense to start gently and progressively to increase the force if needed.

Each manipulation must always be followed by re-assessment.

Traction

Most types of spinal manipulation in orthopedic medicine are performed under traction. Traction facilitates the reduction of a displaced fragment and provides an important safety element against the possibility of a protrusion contacting the spinal cord during manipulation.

Slack

All spinal manipulations are performed over only small amplitude. Therefore, all 'slack' must be taken up by moving the vertebral joints passively to the end of the normal passive range of movement.

Thrust

Immediately after the slack has been taken up in the surrounding tissues, minimal amplitude, high-velocity thrust is given to affect the target tissue.

The amount of force used for the final thrust depends mainly on the patient and manipulator. The length of the lever is also important. The force should always be kept reasonable and may be progressively increased, according to the immediate result.

Leverage

The amount of force used depends on the length of the lever. The longer the lever, the less force is needed.

Reassessment

After each maneuver the patient is assessed, the criteria of success being the absence of symptoms and the restoration of pain-free movement.

We strongly believe that spinal pain is the result of disc protrusion that gives rise to a conflict between the posterocentral or posterolateral rim of the disc and the pain-sensitive dura mater or dural nerve sleeve, and that a displaced fragment of an intervertebral disc can be moved by manipulation. This was the hypothesis of Cyriax.

INJECTION AND INFILTRATION TECHNIQUE

Musculoskeletal disorders such as tendinitis, minor muscular ruptures, ligamentous sprains and arthritis can usually be treated by infiltration. For an optimal effect the product administered must be put directly into the lesion and not in its surroundings. The descriptive terms 'injection' and 'infiltration' are used; each has a well-defined meaning and expresses a different way by which the product is administered. In *injection* the tip of the needle is placed in exactly the right place and all the product is deposited at one single push, as is done in an ordinary intramuscular injection. This technique is mainly used for intra-articular and caudal epidural injections. Local administration of a drug into a structure, as in bursitis, tendinitis, tenosynovitis, tenovaginitis, lesions of a muscle belly and also in ligamentous problems, is usually performed by *infiltration*. In this, maximal beneficial effect is obtained when all the different areas within the lesion receive some of the product. This can only be achieved if the tip of the needle is displaced several times while injecting a small amount of the product at each point. An infiltration is, therefore, a series of injections, given at slightly different places, within the lesion. In orthopedic medicine three types of product are used—local anesthetics, corticosteroids and sclerosant solution.

CHAPTER

6

McKenzie Method of Mechanical Diagnosis and Therapy

Krishna N Sharma

HISTORY

- It was developed by Mr Robin Anthony McKenzie, a physiotherapist from New Zealand born in Auckland in 1931 (Fig. 6.1).
- It was invented in 1956 by accident when one of his backache patients Mr Smith was instructed to lie face down in on the examination table in the treatment room while waiting for Mr McKenzie to come. The room was vacated by a knee patient so the treatment table was elevated. When Mr McKenzie entered in the room and saw the back patient lying in prone position with back extension on that bed, he was shocked as it was believed to be very dangerous position for back pain. Concerned with his wellbeing, Mr McKenzie asked how he and surprisingly Mr Smith replied "This is the best I have felt in three weeks". This incidence forced Mr McKenzie to re-think about whatever he had been taught about spine and pain.

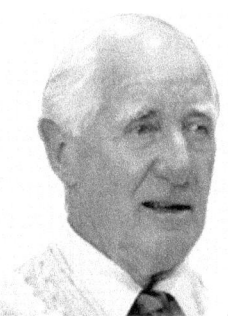

Fig. 6.1: Robin Anthony McKenzie.

- Since the patients used to feel relief in the pain in the extremities and the pain used to remain just in the spinal level and surroundings, it was initially called *centralization*.
- In 1979, he classified the back pain in three classes.
- In 1981, he officially launched mechanical diagnosis and therapy (MDT)—a system encompassing assessment (evaluation), diagnosis and treatment for the spine and extremities.

CONCEPT

- The McKenzie MDT has three steps—*evaluation, treatment* and *prevention*.
- Self-healing and self-treatment are more important for pain rehabilitation. It includes three phases:
  1. Educating and demonstrating patients the relieving and aggravating effects of prescribed movements and harmful movements.
  2. Educating and demonstrating how to maintain the reduced or abolished symptoms.
  3. Educating and demonstrating how to restore full-function without symptoms.

EVALUATION

Though taking history and other necessary physical examination is a part of evaluation to find out the degree of impairment and red flags, what makes MDT evaluation different is finding *centralization* and *directional preference of movement*.

During evaluation, the therapist tries to find a pattern of mechanical and symptomatic responses called *centralization,* i.e. shifting the symptoms centrally (towards mid-back or neck).

To find centralization, the therapist tries to provoke and relieve the symptoms by sustaining the patients in certain positions and or ask to do some end range spinal movements, e.g. flexion, extension, lateral flexion, and combination. The direction of motion that elicits centralization is called *directional preference of movement*. Based on the subjective phenomenon (range of motion, antalgic posturing, etc.) and objective phenomenon (symptom location, frequency, duration, etc.), the patients are classified into three groups name according to pathoanatomical explanations.

CLASSIFICATION

After evaluation, the patients are classified into three groups:
1. Postural syndrome
2. Dysfunctional syndrome
3. Derangement syndrome
   a. Reducible
   b. Irreducible

Postural Syndrome (Normal Tissues-Bad Stress)

It is due to excessive and or prolonged end-range stress on normal tissues, e.g. muscles, tendons, joint, etc. The characteristics of this class are:
- Intermittent pain
- Pain-free full range of motion is available
- Patient complains pain in certain prolonged sustained postures
- Pain is reproduced only in the end-range prolonged loading, e.g. sustained slouched sitting position
- The pain disappears when the patient changes that static position.

Dysfunctional Syndrome (Normal Stress-Short Tissues)

It is due to tissue shortening (scarring, fibrosis, adhesion) or spasm that limit the range of motion and cause pain at the end-range. The characteristics of this class are:
- Loss of range of motion
- Symptoms at the end-range of the movement.

Derangement Syndrome

It is due to anatomical disruption or displacement (e.g. intervertebral disc prolapse) in the normal resting position of the affected joint surfaces. It is further classified into:

Reducible Derangement
- Pain in early end-range
- Stiffness with or without pain
- Symptoms decrease or centralize by repeated movement in one direction, i.e. directional preference
- Repeated movement opposite to directional preference produce, increase or peripheralization the symptoms
- Patient is able to centralizes and maintain centralization.

Irreducible Derangement
  - Features of derangement syndrome
  - No centralization or maintenance of centralization till at least 3–5 sessions.

TREATMENT

The treatment depends upon the type of syndrome.

Postural Syndrome (Respect the Pain… Don't Do if it Hurts)
- Postural correction: It can be done in the following steps:
  - Let the patient sit in provocative sitting posture (slouched).
  - Overcorrect the posture (hyper-extend the lumbar spine and hyper-retract the head and neck simultaneously)
  - Now instruct the patient to let go 10% to find neutral sitting position.
- Avoiding provocative postures.
- Strengthening of postural muscles.

Dysfunctional Syndrome *(No Pain No Gain)*
Mobilizing exercises in the direction of pain remodels the motion limiting tissue. It takes little long time to show effectiveness.

Derangement Syndrome
Treatment according to the clinically induced directional preference.

SEVERITY INDICATORS (LESS SESSIONS NEEDED TO MORE SESSION NEEDED)
- Central of symmetrical symptoms
- Unilateral and asymmetrical symptoms to knee
- Unilateral and asymmetrical symptoms to below knee.

CHAPTER 7

Osteopathy

Krishna N Sharma

HISTORY

The term "osteopathy" was coined by *Andrew Taylor Still*—a physician and surgeon at the time of the American Civil War. In Baldwin, he developed the practice of osteopathy. The practice of osteopathy began in the United States in 1874. *Still* named his new school of medicine Osteopathy, reasoning that the bone, *osteon*, was the starting point from which he was to ascertain the cause of pathological conditions (Fig. 7.1).

Osteopathic medicine represents one of two distinct schools of medicine in the United States.

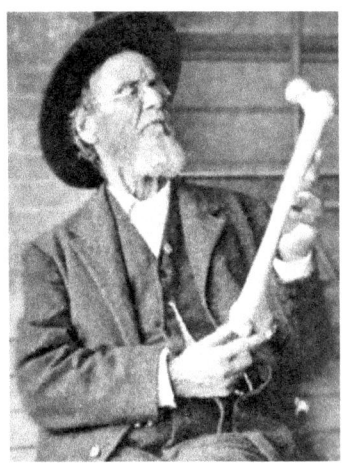

Fig. 7.1: Andrew Taylor Still.

Osteopathy is one of the two groups of fully licensed physicians in the United States. Osteopathic medical institutions issue Doctor of Osteopathic Medicine or Doctor of Osteopathy (DO) degrees, and allopathic medical institutions issue Medical Doctor (MD) degrees.

OSTEOPATHIC PRINCIPLES

These principles by osteopathic physicians are not held to be empirical laws; they serve, rather, as the underpinnings of the osteopathic philosophy on health and disease. There were only four major principles of osteopathic medicine in the beginning but with time, few other principles were added.

The *basic principles of osteopathic philosophy* are:
1. *The body is a unit:* The osteopathy believes that though the body does consist of parts—all work to benefit the organism in totality. Infact the human body does not function as a collection of separate parts but rather as an integral whole.
2. *Structure and function are interrelated:* According to this principle the body structures and functions are interconnected. Any change in one of them affects another. For example, the joint structures like the bony ends, musculature, ligaments, and other periarticular tissues govern the degree of motion and any pathological change in the joint structure will limit the joint function like decreased range of motion and improper weight bearing. At the same time any abnormal motion or limited motion at the joint will change the joint structures which may be seen as the shortening or abnormal lengthening of the ligaments, muscle atrophy, and cartilage degeneration, etc.
3. *The body possesses self-regulatory mechanisms:* Our body itself regulates all its functions. For example, the baroreceptors and carotid sinus monitor blood pressure and regulates the heart rate according to that. Our body uses the nervous system, and endocrine system, etc. to regulate itself.
4. *Rational treatment is based on applying these principles:* The osteopathic treatment is formulated by applying these principles with the association of anatomy and physiology.
5. *The body has the inherent capacity to defend and repair itself:* The body has capability to defend itself from the various micro/macro-organisms and repair itself after injury. The skin, nasal mucus and hairs, etc. are just few of the examples of its defensive structures. After any injury like fracture, we immobilize the bone to prevent any further injury, but it is the body only which repairs the bone.
6. *When normal adaptability is disrupted, or when environmental changes overcome the body's capacity for self-maintenance, disease may ensue:* Any disease occurs either when the adverse environmental factors overcome the body's defenses, or when the body is not able to adapt to a situation.

Apart from these principles, there are few corollary principles also:
1. *Movement of body fluids is essential to the maintenance of health:* Any disturbance in the fluid circulation produces pathology,

Osteopathy

or delay the healing process. Because of this it is advisable to focus on areas of dysfunction that influence the circulation to an affected area.

2. *The nervous system plays a crucial part in controlling the body:* The nervous system plays very important role in controlling the movement of body fluids. So the osteopaths focus on resume the normal autonomic tone to correct the vascular response.
3. *There are somatic components to disease that not only are manifestations of disease but also are factors that contribute to maintenance of the diseased state:* Any direct injury to the neuromusculoskeletal structure, or any response of viscera to pathology may cause the somatic component of the disease process.

TECHNIQUES OF OSTEOPATHIC TREATMENT

Osteopathic manipulative treatment (OMT) is the therapeutic application of manually guided forces by an osteopathic physician to improve physiologic function and/or support homeostasis that has been altered by somatic dysfunction.

There are numerous OMTs which are classified in the following way:

Direct Treatment Modalities

In the direct method, the osteopath thrusts the restricted joint or tissue through the restrictive barrier in the direction of the restriction to motion. The direct treatment modalities include:
- Soft tissue techniques
- Articulatory treatment system
- High velocity low amplitude (HVLA)
- Muscle energy technique
- Inhibition.

Indirect Treatment Modalities

In the indirect method, the osteopath positions the joint or tissue away from the barrier to motion setting up the tissues to "unwind" and move through the restrictive barrier on its own.
- Articulatory technique
- Balanced ligamentous tension

- Balanced membranous tension
- Craniosacral
- Energy engaging
- Facilitated positional release
- Functional indirect
- Indirect myofascial release
- Manual percussion and vibration
- Nerve release
- Strain/counter-strain
- Visceral manipulation.

Combined Treatment Modalities

The combined techniques include both the direct and indirect components. There are various combinations of the techniques mentioned in the above two categories. Apart from that, few techniques mentioned above are modified and that is why they may fall in this category also. One of the combined treatment modality is *Still Technique*.

Treatment Modalities that are neither Direct nor Indirect

There are few techniques which do not fall in any of the above categories. Few of them are:
- Chapman's reflexes
- Lymphatic techniques.

CHAPTER 8

Chiropractic

Kuki Bordoloi

The term *Chiropractic* came from the Greek words *cheir (hand)* and *praxis (practice)* to describe a treatment done by hand. It is a form of alternative medicine which is concerned with the diagnosis, treatment and prevention of mechanical disorders of the neuro-musculoskeletal system. Though most of the controlled clinical studies and systemic reviews have not found it very effective in the cases other than the neck pain, back pain, etc.; and most important—it is not a part of physiotherapy, I thought

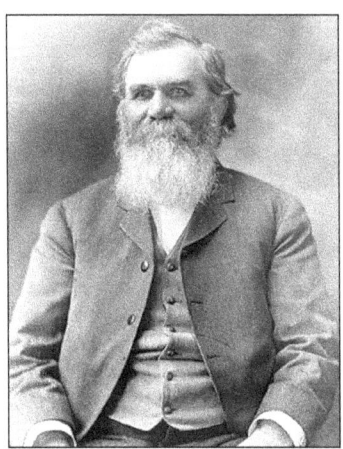

Fig. 8.1: DD Palmer.

to put it in this text so that the students may differentiate between the manual therapy and chiropractic. Chiropractic, believe that spine problems disturbs the body's general functions and innate intelligence, a notion that brings criticism from mainstream health care. *Daniel David Palmer* who was a magnetic healer in Iowa is the father of Chiropractic (Fig. 8.1). He founded in the 1895, and later his son *BJ Palmer* expanded it in the early 20th century. Traditional chiropractic was based on the vitalism, but with time they adapted conventional medical techniques, such as massage, exercise, heat therapy, and cryotherapy, etc. Due to the emphasis on the vitalism, the chiropractors faced strong opposition from the medical community and thousands of chiropractors including *DD Palmer* were prosecuted for practicing medicine without a license and were jailed. Later to protect themselves from the jurisdiction, *BJ Palmer* argued that they were distinct from medicine, as they "analyzed" rather than "diagnosed", and "adjusted" subluxations rather than "treated" disease.

PHILOSOPHY OF CHIROPRACTIC

The Chiropractic is based on both the materialistic and vitalistic belief. The materialistic belief is based on the concept that since the spinal misalignment causes the disorders, the chiropractic adjustment will improve the health condition because of the restoration of structural integrity. The vitalistic belief says that interruptions in the flow of innate intelligence, a vital nervous energy or life force—affect the body physiology. However, the chiropractic philosophy includes the following perspectives:

- *Holism:* It believes that everything in an individual's environment may affect the health. It covers even the spiritual and existential dimension.
- *Reductionism:* It believes that the vertebral subluxation is the cause of health problems and only it is mandatory to reduce the subluxation in order to cure the problem.
- *Conservatism:* It avoids medication and surgery to minimize risk of clinical interventions and emphasizes noninvasive conservative management.
- *Homeostasis:* It emphasizes the body's inherent self-healing abilities.

This diversity in the belief system has divided the Chiropractors in two groups—*Straight Chiropractors*, and *Mixed Chiropractors*.

Straight Chiropractors

Straight chiropractors are vitalistics and rely only on the philosophical principles by DD and BJ Palmer. They believe that vertebral subluxation interferes with an "innate intelligence" exerted via the human nervous system and it causes diseases. They do not feel the necessity of the medical diagnosis and are mainly concerned with the detection and correction of vertebral subluxation.

Mixed Chiropractors

They believe that subluxation is not only but actually one of the causes of disease and that is why they mix chiropractic with the medical and osteopathic diagnostic and treatment approaches.

TREATMENT TECHNIQUES

The chiropractors apply dynamic *high-velocity, low-amplitude spinal manipulation (HVLA-SM)* thrusts to manipulate the spine to which they call *Chiropractic Adjustment*. The chiropractors mixed different techniques from different chiropractic school as within this time period of more than a century, more than 100 techniques are developed by different chiropractors. Few of them are:

- Access seminars *(by Weignat, Blooment)*
- Activator technique *(by Lee, Fuhr)*
- Adjustive instrument
- Alternative chiropractic adjustments *(by Wiehe)*
- Applied chiropractic distortion analysis *(by Kotheimer)*
- Applied kinesiology *(by Goodheart, Walters, Schmitt, Thie)*
- Applied spinal biomechanical engineering *(by Aragona)*
- Aquarian age healing *(by Hurley)*
- Arnholz muscle adjusting *(by Arnholz)*
- Atlas orthogonality technique *(by Sweat)*
- Atlas specific *(by Wernsing)*
- Bandy seminars *(by Bandy)*
- Bio-kinesiology *(by Barton)*
- Bio-energetic synchronization technique *(by Morter)*
- Bioenergetics *(by Broeringmeyer)*
- Biomagnetic technique *(by Stoffels, Borham, Broeringmeyer)*
- Blair upper cervical technique *(by Blair)*
- Bloodless surgery *(by Lorenz, Failor, DeJarnette)*
- Body integration *(by Espy)*
- Buxton technical course of painless chiropractic *(by Buxton)*
- CHOKE system *(by Johnson)*
- Chiro plus kinesiology *(by Dowty)*
- Chiroenergetics *(by Kimmel)*
- Chirometry *(by Quigly)*
- Chiropractic concept *(by Prill)*
- Chiropractic manipulative reflex technique *(by DeJarnette)*
- Chiropractic neuro-biomechanical analysis
- Chiropractic spinal biophysics *(by Harrison)*
- Clinical kinesiology *(by Beardall)*
- Collins method of painless adjusting *(by Collins)*
- Concept therapy *(by Fleet, Dill)*
- Cox/flexion-distraction

- Cranial the chnique *(by DeJarnette, Goodheart)*
- Craniopathy *(by Cottam)*
- Directional non-force technique *(by Van Rumpt, Johns)*
- Distraction technique *(by James Cox)*
- Diversified technique *(by Bonyun, Carver, Crawford, DeGiacomo, Grecco, Lebeau, Metzinger, Reinert, States, Stonebrink, Stierwalt)*
- Endo-nasal technique *(by Gibbons, Lake, Broeringmeyer)*
- Extremity technique *(by Schultz)*
- Focalizer spinal recoil *(by George)*
- Freeman chiropractic procedure *(by Freeman)*
- Fundamental chiropractic *(by Ashton)*
- Global energetic matrix *(by Babinet)*
- Gonstead technique *(by Gonstead)*
- Grostic *(by Grostic)*
- Herring cervical technique *(by Herring)*
- Holographic diagnosis and treatment *(by Franks, Gleason)*
- Howard system *(by Howard)*
- Keck method of analysis *(by Keck)*
- King tetrahedron concept *(by King)*
- Lemond brainstem technique *(by Lemond)*
- Logan basic technique *(by Logan, Coggins)*
- Master energy dynamics *(by Bartlett)*
- Mawhiney scoliosis technique *(by Mawhiney)*
- McTimody technique *(by McTimody)*
- Mears technique *(by Mears)*
- Medicine-assisted manipulation
- Meric technique system *(by Cleveland, BJ Palmer, Loban, Forster, Riley)*
- Micromanipulation *(by Young)*
- Motion palpation *(by Gillet)*
- Muscle palpation *(by Spano)*
- Muscle response testing *(by Lepore, Fishman, Grinims)*
- Musculoskeletal synchronization and stabilization technique *(by Krippenbrock)*
- Nerve signal interference *(by Craton)*
- Network chiropractic *(by Epstein)*
- Neuro-emotional technique *(by Walker)*
- Neuro-organizational technique *(by Ferrari)*

- Neuro-lymphatic reflex technique *(by Chapman)*
- Neurovascular reflex technique *(by Bennett)*
- Nimmo receptor-tonus technique
- Oleshy 21st century technique *(by Olesky)*
- Ortman technique *(by Ortman)*
- Perianal posture reflex technique *(by Watkins)*
- Pettibon spinal biomechanics technique *(by Pettibon)*
- Pierce-Stillwagon technique *(by Pierce, Stillwagon)*
- Polarity technique
- Posture imbalance patterns *(by Sinclaire)*
- Pure chiropractic technique *(by Morreim)*
- Reaver's 5th cervical key *(by Reaver, Pierce)*
- Receptor tonus technique *(by Nimmo)*
- Riddler reflex technique *(by Riddler)*
- Sacro-occipital technique *(by DeJarnette)*
- Soft tissue orthopedics *(by Rees)*
- Somatosynthesis *(by Ford)*
- Spears painless system *(by Spears)*
- Specific majors *(by Nemiroff)*
- Spinal stress/stressology *(by Ward)*
- Spinal touch technique *(by Rosquist)*
- Spondylotherapy *(by Forster, Riley)*
- Stimulus reflex effector technique
- Thompson terminal point technique *(by Thompson)*
- Tieszen technique *(by Tieszen)*
- Toftness technique *(by Toftness)*
- Top notch viseral techniques *(by Portelli, Marcellino)*
- Tortipelvis/torticollis *(by Barge)*
- Total body modification *(by Frank)*
- Touch for health *(by Thie)*
- Truscott technique *(by Truscott)*
- Ungerank specific low force chiropractic technique *(by Ungerank)*
- Upper cervical technique/HIO, Toggle *(by BJ Palmer, Duff,* Kale, Life College, NUCCA)
- Variable force technique *(by Leighton)*
- Von Fox combination technique *(by Von Fox)*
- Zindler reflex technique *(by Zindl)*

The mixed chiropractors use the following measures also which are adapted from physiotherapy and other health professions:
- ADL management
- Cryotherapy
- Ergonomics
- Heat therapy
- Nutritional and dietary recommendations
- Postural correction
- Relaxation techniques
- Therapeutic exercise
- Trigger point therapy

CHAPTER 9

Krishna's Kinetikinetic Manual Therapy®

Krishna N Sharma

Krishna's Kinetikinetic Manual Therapy® (KKMT®) is a school of thought in manual therapy founded by Dr Krishna N Sharma, a physiotherapist from India. KKMT® emphasizes on realigning the incongruity or recoiling the restrictions of joint by mobilization and manipulation to facilitate the homeostatic kinetic forces of joint.

HISTORY

- The concept of KKMT® Mobilization (3D Glides®) first sprouted in 2004 when I was still a student.
- The first draft of basic concepts and techniques for knee joint KKMT® completed on September 4th, 2015.
- The first 2 students who learned KKMT® for knee joint were *Mr Donfack Philip* (Assistant Lecturer at St Louis University, Cameroon) and *Mr Chu Buh Franklin* (student under University of Rome Tor Vergata, Italy)
- The first batch of KKMT® mobilization (knee joint) was taught on the 19th of March, 2016 in St Louis University Campus, Cameroon.
- This first ever book on KKMT® was published in April, 2016.
- The KKMT® was introduced in the national physiotherapy curriculum of the Ministry of Higher Education, Cameroon (Africa).
- This first two researchers who evaluated the effectiveness of KKMT® were *Miss Foyet Azongmo Lolita* and *Miss Diang Hilda Ngwe*.

PRINCIPLES

The KKMT® joint mobilization techniques are based on the following principles:
1. Proper arthrokinematic motion and homeostatic kinetic forces are essential for proper and smooth osteokinematic motion.

2. Homeostatic kinetics of the joint is important to maintain static and dynamic alignment of a joint. The homeostatic kinetic forces help the joint come back in its proper alignment after a motion. The factors that produce and govern the homeostatic kinetics of joint are:
   a. Local/intrinsic factors, e.g. ligament, cartilage, meniscus, etc.
   b. Global/extrinsic factors, e.g. muscles, fascia, gravity, etc.
3. Limitation or restrictions in the arthrokinematic motion can be restored by facilitating homeostatic kinetics of the intrinsic and extrinsic factors.

INDICATIONS
- Joint pain
- Decreased range of motion (ROM).

CONTRAINDICATIONS
Though pain during application of the techniques itself is the best way to know if the technique is contraindicated, KKMT® joint mobilization should be applied with caution in the cases of acute injuries, e.g. fracture, acute sprain, etc. and joint instability.

TECHNIQUES
The KKMT® joint mobilization is applied after muscle and joint conditioning. There is a range to techniques that can be applied to restore the joint motion and facilitate the homeostatic kinetics. Few of them are below:
i. Joint Gaping®
ii. 3D Gliding®
iii. Functional Articular Rolling®

Joint Gaping®
It is a joint distraction technique performed with functional osteo-kinematic motion.

Functional 3D Gliding®
There is never a unidirectional arthrokinematic motion in a functional joint, so I started exploring the possibilities of 3D gliding and

coined the term—3D Glide®. The restricted/painful osteokinematic movement is performed passively with variations of 3D glide patterns to identify the preferred pattern.

Since physiologically, 3D glides occur obviously only during active motion and not when the joint is static, I prefer to perform the 3D glides only with active motion. The 3D Glide® patterns can be combined with other techniques, e.g. post-isometric relaxation, reciprocal inhibition, oculocervical reflex, etc. too.

Functional Articular Rolling®

Rolling is the most ignored component in manual therapy as most of the techniques focus on gliding only. My joint rolling techniques are mostly combined with joint gaping®.

CHAPTER

10

Translatoric Spinal Manipulation™

Krishna N Sharma

Translatoric spinal manipulation (TSM) consists of a series of high and low velocity manipulative spinal techniques.

HISTORY

It was developed by Olaf Evjenth PT, OMT in collaboration with Freddy Kaltenborn PT, OMT (Fig. 10.1).

CONCEPT

This technique is useful in the cases of spinal hypomobility. The patient is diagnosed with the help of history, observation of active motions and passive angular and translatoric motion testing. This technique is used only when the patient is diagnosed with spinal hypomobility.

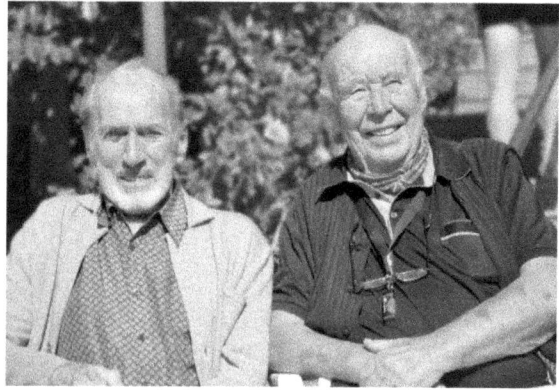

Fig. 10.1: Olaf Evjenth and Freddy Kaltenborn.

In this technique, the therapist uses small amplitude and straight line (iranslatoric) traction or gliding impulses which is delivered parallel or at a right angle of an individual vertebral joint or movement segment. Direct manual stabilization or spinal pre-positioning is also used to restrict the motion at other spinal segments during the treatment to localize the effects.

HYPOTHESIZED MECHANISMS BEHIND EFFECTS

1. **Mechanical:**
   a. Stretching of peri-articular tissues
   b. Releasing trapped intra-articular meniscoids
   c. Breaking of tissue adhesion
   d. Restoration of gliding within fascial planes.
2. **Neurological:**
   a. Stimulation of mechanoceptors
   b. Change in pain perception
   c. Change in resting muscle tone.
3. **Hydraulic:** Change in synovial fluid viscosity and distribution.
4. **Circulatory:** Reduction of circulatory congestion due to reduction in pressure in the intervertebral foramen and muscle tissues.
5. **Psychological:** Placebo effect.

TECHNIQUES

- **Disc traction:** *It is applied at a right angle to the surface of the disc joint. It decompresses the disc and intervertebral foramen.*
- **Facet distraction:** *In this technique, the spinal segment is positioned in side bending and rotation in opposite directions.*
- **Facet gliding:** *This technique is applied with the spinal segment in a coupled position. Gliding is perform parallel to the articular surface and adjacent spinal segments are stabilized through direct manual contact or through spinal locking.*

CHAPTER 11

Matos Maneuver

Krishna N Sharma

Matos maneuver is a manual therapy technique created by Nuno Matos in 1997 and registered in 2002. The Matos maneuver was presented in Estoril on the 1st International Congress of the Portuguese Association of Physiotherapists—Manual Therapy Special Interest Group (IFOMT-ECE) 2002 and in Barcelona on the 14th International WCPT Congress 2003.

THEORETICAL BASIS

This maneuver is based on an adaptation of the long sitting with the application of a cranial handle, with the aim of simultaneous lengthening of all chains, neuromeningeal, posterior muscular chain and miomeningeal chain. It allows to focus on the structures and fascia aponeurosis, since the insertion of the suboccipital muscles, more precisely, smaller posterior rectus muscle of head is at the dura mater. Since it is very effective in any shrinkage of the 3 chains, it seems to be better than other techniques when it comes to achieve higher mobility.

TECHNIQUE

The patient sits on the treatment table in long sitting position keeping the knees extended and ankles off the edge of the table. The arms are placed behind the back in relaxed position with the palms facing upward. The patient performs active flexion of the neck.

Now the therapist holds the head of the patients using *cranial handle*. The therapist places both the palms in such a way that the thumbs are on the cranial vault, the second and third fingers encircle the ear and the fourth and fifth fingers are on the anterolateral surface.

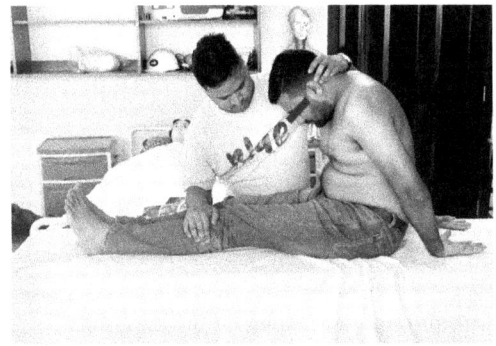

Fig. 11.1: Therapist performing Matos maneuver.

The therapist now applies little amount of force for passive flexion and instructs the patients to do plantar and dorsiflexion of the ankle.

It is recommended to perform two-three sets of three repetitions (Fig. 11.1).

CONTRAINDICATIONS
- Acute cervical disc pathology
- Arnold-Chiari syndrome
- Cervical spine instability
- Injuries of the upper cervical spine
- Osteoporosis
- Respiratory problems
- Vertebrobasilar syndrome.

CHAPTER 12

Visceral Manipulation

Krishna N Sharma

Visceral manipulation (VM) was developed by a French Osteopath and Physical Therapist Jean-Pierre Barral. He started teaching VM in 1985 (Fig. 12.1).

INTRODUCTION

Though it is well known that Dr Still used few techniques to the viscera, but he never documented that what he did. But *Dr Barral* worked on it and developed his own techniques of visceral manipulation.

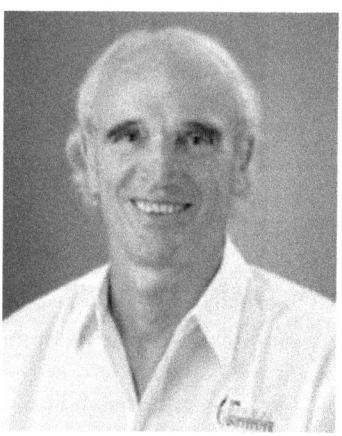

Fig. 12.1: Jean-Pierre Barral.

BASICS

Dr Barral observed two visceral phenomena:
1. *Mobility:* It is gross movement of the viscera within the abdomen, e.g. peristaltic motion of intestine. It is believed to occur due to pressure changes, changes in the ligamentous support system, muscular activity, and articulatory changes with regard to adjacent viscera.

   Mobility can be restricted due to the flowing causes:
   - Ligamentous system restrictions due to adhesions or laxity resulting in organ ptosis.
   - Intracavitary pressure restrictions due to diaphragmatic dysfunction or turgor abnormalities.
   - Organ restrictions due to adhesions.
   - Double layer system abnormalities due to fluid restrictions, i.e. pleurisy.
   - Muscular restrictions via viscerospasms and vice versa.

2. *Motility:* It is inherent small motions particular to individual organs. It is inherent motion generated within the organ itself. It is theorized to be a repetition of the embryologic unfolding of the organ. The rate of visceral motility is believed to be on the 6-8 cycles per minute and the amplitude is believed to be approximately 500 microns to several millimeters of excursion. Motility is further explained by the terms *expire* and *inspire*.
   - Expire—motion toward midline.
   - Inspire—motion away from midline.

   Motility restrictions also cause diseases or disorders. All organs will have a propensity for either expire or inspire and this does not necessarily indicate dysfunction. Dysmotility can be defined as an overwhelming propensity for either phase, abnormalities within a given plane of its 3-dimensional motility, or a ratcheting motion during a particular phase.

INDICATIONS

The indications are following but not limited to:
- Cardiac conditions
- Respiratory conditions
- Gastrointestinal conditions
- Endocrine disorders
- Urogenital conditions.

CONTRAINDICATIONS

- Recent surgery
- Inflamed organ
- Infected organ
- Bleeding organ
- Suspicion of abdominal etiologies requiring medical clearance
- Skin lesions wherein pressure is intolerable.

DIAGNOSIS

It can be done with the concepts of biomechanics or separately as a global fascial, regional fascial, or local listening diagnosis.
- *Global listening:* Identifying the key lesion via palpation of fascial tension.
- *Local listening:* Closer inspection near the area identified with global listening.

- *Thermal evaluation:* It is another option to evaluate for the key lesion through the energy.

TECHNIQUES AND STYLES

The techniques are classified into three categories:
1. Direct
2. Indirect
3. Combined

The styles are classified into:
- Alleviation of somatic dysfunction
- Reflex oriented
- Myofascial oriented
- Balanced ligamentous tension/ligamentous articular strain
- Vibratory/stimulatory technique.

CHAPTER 13

Strain Counterstrain

Harshita Yadav

DEFINITIONS

It is defined as "passive positional procedure that places the body in a position of greatest comfort, thereby relieving pain by reduction and arrest of inappropriate proprioceptive activity that maintain somatic dysfunction".
—**Lawrence Jones (1981)**

It is a passive positional aimed at relieving musculoskeletal pain and dysfunction through indirect manual manipulation also known as positional release therapy (PRT) which is a derivative form of Jones' strain counterstrain (SCS).
—**D' Ambrogio and Roth (1997)**

HISTORY

SCS is the fourth most commonly used osteopathic manipulative technique followed by soft tissue techniques, high velocity low amplitude thrust, and muscle energy technique.

In 1981, Jones' by his clinical experience charted over 200 specific tender points which are related to particular strain patterns (flexion, extension) and structure (ligaments, muscles, joints). First observation made by Jones' in for both acute and chronic strain was the position of comfort or ease with a hold of 90 seconds to that tissue which are already shortened by giving support in even a shorter state, allowing neurological and circulatory mechanism to operate in resolution of dysfunction state.

George Goodheart (in Walther 1988) described a universally applicable formula which relies more on individual features displayed by patient and less on rigid recipes used in Jones' and less on PRT therapy and approaches. He suggests that a suitable tender point should be searched in opposite tissues which are "active" during pain or restriction. He concluded that if a facilitating crowding or neuromuscular manipulation of spindle is utilized, a 20-30 seconds hold of the position of ease is adequate.

ADVANTAGES
- Point will relate specifically to individual's problem which is located in response to identified pain or restriction.
- Number of tender points can be evaluated because there are variety of movements which may produce pain or restriction.
- By means of *"self-treatment and self-aid"* this concept can effectively used in chronic pain condition where patient are taught within few minutes to achieve a pain relieving condition for significant periods.

McPartland and Zigler (1993) give another concept according to which the therapist will be able to treat any painful tissue using positional release, is valid whether the pain is being monitored via feedback from the patient or whether the concept of assessing a reduction in tone in tissues is being used. A lengthening period up to 90 seconds is recommended for holding the position for maximum ease.

Schiowitz (1990) described the position of distressed area into the direction of its greatest freedom of moment, starting from a position of *"neutral"* in terms of overall body position. He states that "the order of two steps, first placing tissue into its position of ease and then applying the force, may be reversed. The mechanism involved is thought to be related to medications and neutral activity which reduces hypertonicity. He also reduces the time for hold to 5 seconds when employing facilitated positional release.

D' Ambrogio and Roth (1997) coined the term PRT which is a derivative of Jones' SCS. The most important element is systematic scanning for the tender points which are assessed prior to treatment. The goal is spend more time on evaluation and less time on treatment which is based on the fact that if most dominant point of the body is located and treated, a majority of other tender points will be eliminated. He suggests that between 1 and 20 minutes may be needed to achieve fascial release.

Leon Chaitow (1996) be noted suggest that the times suggested above are approximate at best, since tissues respond are approximate at best, since tissues respond idiosyncratically, depending on multiple factors, tissue released should be noted. He also supported the hold for 90 seconds as minimum time for the treatment.

PHYSIOLOGY

SCS is an *indirect technique* because its action is away from restriction barrier. The position of ease often equals the position of strain—so that the patient need to go back in a slow motion, until tenderness vanishes from a tender point which was being monitored, and/or until a sense of ease was perceived in the previously hypertonic shortened tissues. This technique is directed towards—aberrant neuromuscular reflexes within tissue not towards tissue injury or damage.

Mechanism in intervention of SCS includes aberrant neuromuscular activity mediated by muscle spindles and local circulation or inflammatory reactions influenced by sympathetic nervous system. Aberrant neuromuscular activity between agonist and antagonist, known as *proprioceptive theory,* through which rapid stretching injury stimulates muscle spindles causing reflexive agonist muscle contraction that resists further stretching. A reflexive counter-contraction resulting from pain induced withdrawal quickly reverses the aggravating movement thereby exciting antagonist muscle spindle. This theory is based on neurophysiologic regulation

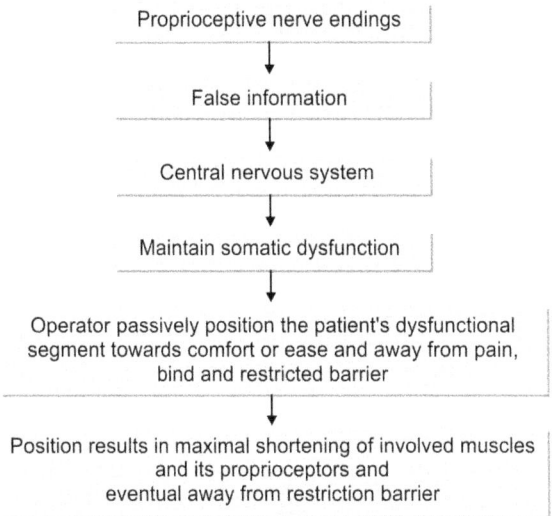

of muscle spindle activity that increases spindle activity and reflexive muscle contraction upon lengthening and decreases spindle discharge and reflexive contraction upon shortening. With passive shortening of the dysfunctional agonist muscle long enough, SCS allows normal muscle spindle activity to return. Once agonist muscle spindle activity is reset, antagonist muscle spindle activity can also return to resting state, relying aberrant neuromuscular activity and restoring normal function.

SCS gave birth to myofacial tender points which are the diagnostic tools of Jones' found by moderate palpatory pressure and directly related to somatic dysfunction. *Tender points are defines as "Small zones of tense, tender, edematous muscle and fascial tissue about a centimeter in diameter".* These tender points are four times more tender than normal tissue.

APPLICATION
Indications
- Alleviating pain
- Enhancing mobility
- Resolution of actual dysfunctional conditions
- Pancreatitis
- Abdominal pain
- Cavus foot
- Cervicothoracic pain
- Complex regional pain syndrome
- Painful and restricted muscles and joints irrespective of cause
- Degenerative spinal and joint conditions, including arthritis
- Post-surgical pain and dysfunction
- Osteoporosis
- Post-traumatic pain and dysfunction, such as sporting injuries, whiplash, ankle sprain, etc.
- Fibromyalgia pain
- Headache
- Pediatric conditions such as torticollis
- Respiratory conditions which might benefit from normalization of primary and accessory breathing muscles, ribs and thoracic spinal restrictions
- Musculoskeletal dysfunctions (like foot, lower back, knee, shoulder)

- Neurological conditions such as dysfunction following cerebral vascular accidents (stroke), spinal or brain injury or degenerative neutral conditions such as multiple sclerosis.

Contraindications and Precautions
- Care should be taken in application of SCS in cases of malignancy, aneurysm and acute inflammatory conditions.
- Skin conditions should be thoroughly assessed thoroughly before the treatment so that undesirable pressure to the tender points could be avoided.
- Protective spasm should not be treated unless the underlying conditions are well considered (like osteoporosis, bone secondaries, disc herniation, fractures, etc).
- Recent major trauma or surgery precludes anything other than gentle superficial positional release methods.
- Infectious conditions call for caution and care.
- Any increase in pain during the positioning shows the undesirable direction, movement or position which need to be cease off. Any sensation like numbness or aching may arise during the positioning of ease or comfort which should be continued until the sensation is moderate and not severe. Also patient should be encouraged to relax and view sensation as transient and part of desirable changes taking place.
- Care should be taken while positioning the patient neck into extension. It is necessary to maintain a periodic communication with the patient along with which the patient is instructed to keep the eyes open so that any signs of nystagmus are observable.

JONES' TECHNIQUE

SCS treatment begins with assessment of specific tender or trigger points to be monitored during and after treatment. The practitioner passively moves the patient into position of comfort while monitoring the tender point. This position should be such that the tenderness should reduce to 70%. The key to successful normalization via the method is attaining the maximum ease of joint, in which the tender point becomes markedly less sensitive to palpation pressure. The practitioner supports the patient in position of comfort for 90 seconds after which the patient is made to return to neutral start position, in order to avoid ballistic proprioceptors firing and restoring the dysfunctional pattern which has just released. Patients are given advised not to do any strenuous activity over the following days. Reassessment of tender points should indicate a reduction in previous sensitivity up to two-third. Post-treatment soreness is a common phenomenon and patients should be told about this prior to the treatment and it will pass over the next 48 hours with or without the attention.

GUIDELINES

The four keys which a therapist needs which allow them to apply the SCS technique efficiently
1. An ability to localize by palpation soft tissue changes related to particular strain dysfunctions, acute or chronic.
2. An ability to sense tissue change as it moves into a state of ease, comfort, relaxation and reduced resistance.
3. The ability to guide the patient as a whole, or the affected body part, towards a state of ease with minimal force.
4. The ability to apply minimal palpation force as the changes in the tissues are evaluated.

The guidelines which should be remembered and applied are:
- Locate and palpate the appropriate tender point
- Use minimal force
- Use minimal monitoring pressure
- Achieve maximum ease/comfort
- Produce no additional pain anywhere else.

CHAPTER 14

Facilitated Positional Release

Kedar K Mate

DEFINITIONS

Facilitated positional release (FPR) is a system of indirect myofascial release treatment in which the component region of the body is placed into a neutral position, diminishing tissue and joint tension in all planes and an activating force (compression or torsion) is added.

It is a functional technique wherein an indirect treatment approach that involves finding the dynamic balance point of one of the following and involves applying an indirect guiding force, holding the position or adding compression to exaggerate position and allow for spontaneous readjustment.

HISTORY

This technique is developed by Stanley Schiowitz, DO in 1990, 'Facilitated Positional Release' in Journal of American Osteopathic Association.

INDICATIONS

- Acute or chronic somatic dysfunctions
- As primary treatment or in conjunction with other approaches
- Muscle spasticity

RELATIVE CONTRAINDICATIONS

- Patient who cannot voluntarily relax
- Severely ill patient
- Severe osteoporosis
- Cervical spine compression can mimic a Spurling maneuver and produce cervical radiculopathy. Treatment can be adapted by using a traction facilitating force instead of compression

- Lumbar discogenic technique contraindicated following hip replacement when external rotation and torque may disarticulate the joint
- Patients should be given usual post-treatment instructions for possible transient fatigue or discomfort related to restoration of circulation to previously dysfunctional tissues.

ABSOLUTE CONTRAINDICATIONS
- Lack of patient consent and/or cooperation
- Absence of somatic dysfunction
- Unstable fracture.

IMPORTANT POINTS
1. Spine is neutral in position. In the cervical spine, a neutral spine position usually involves a reduction in the usual lordosis. Spine in neutral position, as defined by Fryette, is the position of any area of the spine in which the facets are idling in the position between the beginning of flexion and the beginning of extension.
2. Uses of a facilitating force usually compression, torsion or a combination of two. Occasionally traction force could also be used.
3. The force is directed to muscle unit involved in somatic dysfunction. FRT is adapted for application to rib and extremities.

MECHANISM OF EFFECT
- The force is directed and intended to act on muscle spindle gamma loop (Fig. 14.1)
- The decrease in gamma motor gain to the muscle spindle results in decreased reactivity to stretch stimuli and elimination of the reflex activation of the alpha motor neuron at the spinal cord
- This results in resetting of the tension and hypertonicity of the extrafusal muscle fibers
- According to Carew a sudden decease in load, the spindles on the muscle become unloaded and the Ia fiber discharges from these spindles cease and no longer excite motor neurons controlling the extrafusal muscle fiber leading to relaxation and lengthening of the muscle.

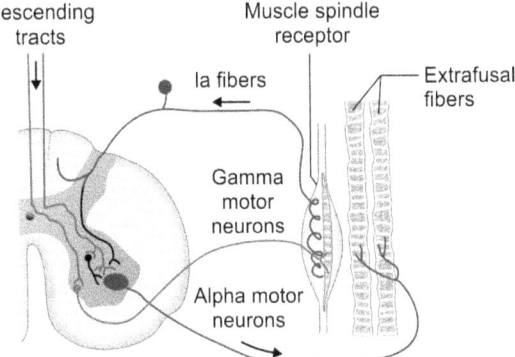

Fig. 14.1: Muscle spindle gamma loop.

- FPR possibly decreases the gain on the muscle spindle and decrease the afferent Ia and II fiber discharges to the motor neurons controlling the extrafusal muscle fiber.

BENEFITS OF FPR
- Normalize hypertonic muscles both superficial and deep.
- Rapid non-traumatic treatment to an affected region
- Easy application for subsequent treatment
- It can be incorporated in any part during a therapy session (initial treatment, subsequent treatment following soft tissue release etc.) and also combined with other treatment techniques.

APPLICATION
- Treatment in most regions can be applied in a seated, supine, prone, or side-lying position
- The physician modifies the patient's sagittal posture in the region to be treated
- A facilitating force is applied (some cases, the position of ease is attained before the facilitating force is applied)
- The large muscle is shortened or the somatic dysfunction is placed into its freedoms of motion
- The position is held for 5 seconds

- This technique could be repeated if the desired results are not achieved
- Release the position and re-evaluate.

MODIFICATIONS TO FRT
- Addition of a direct component of treatment, moving in the barrier directions similar to Still technique as described by van Buskirk
- Addition of "jiggling", a type of microarticulatory oscillation directed to the segment being treated.

CHAPTER 15

Instrument Assisted Soft Tissue Mobilization

Mohamed Kassim Abdul Wahab

INTRODUCTION

Instrument assisted soft tissue mobilization or simply IASTM is a new range of tool (Figs. 15.1 to 15.3) which enables clinicians to efficiently locate and treat individuals diagnosed with soft tissue dysfunction. It is performed with ergonomically designed instruments that detect and treat fascial restrictions, encourage rapid localization and effectively treat areas exhibiting soft tissue fibrosis, chronic inflammation, or degeneration.

HISTORY

Though IASTM is a relatively new technique, it is considered to be a modern evolution from Traditional Chinese Medicine called "Gua Sha" which originated from Asia. However, Gua Sha was not used to treat Musculoskeletal conditions but was traditionally applied

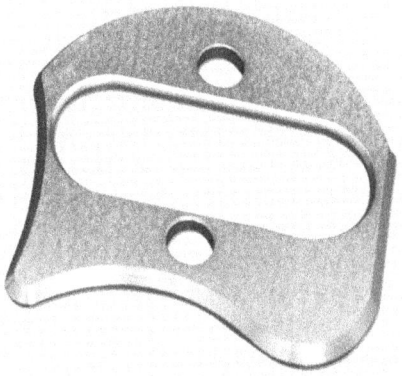

Fig. 15.1: Edge tool.

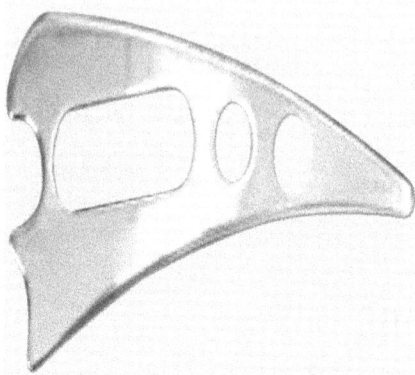

Fig. 15.2: M2T blade.

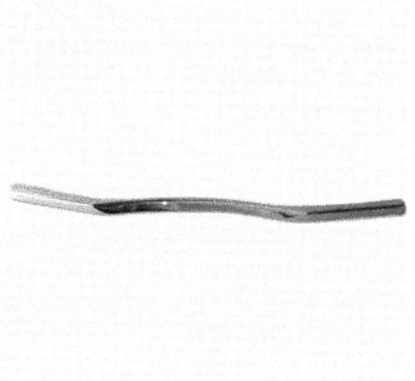

Fig. 15.3: Handlebar.

along meridiens as a means to move stagnant blood from the tissues without it escaping from the skin. More importantly, "Gua Sha" included palpation and cutaneous stimulation over compressed areas of the body with rounded objects, such as spoons, coins, and pieces of water buffalo horns to promote normal circulation and metabolic processes. The manifestation from this modality was redness of the skin, known as "sha," believed to have let out bad "chi." This ancient technique is still used today, and allows for blood flow within and around subcutaneous soft-tissue, enabling circulation and metabolic functioning. Though Gua Sha technique is not used in modern soft tissue therapy, this theory and modality has led to more recent, but traditional, approaches to instrument-assisted soft tissue mobilization.

The current use of instruments in soft tissue mobilization was developed in 1987. David Graston a machinist suffered a knee injury, leaving him in need of reconstructive surgery. When traditional rehabilitation failed to help with his post-surgical scar tissue, he developed the tools, which provided a remarkable improvement of his scar tissue. This led him to experiment on a variety of conditions. Initially the treatment approach was based on Cyriax's soft tissue treatments involving frictions, moving on to the use of mechanical loading principles and recently dwelling into neurophysiological principles. These instruments were modeled from wood, then aluminum when it was introduced. However, stainless steel is currently used as the material of choice.

HOW DOES IT WORK?

IASTM has several effects on body systems. It helps to restore optimal soft tissue quality by causing controlled micro-trauma to the specified area, stimulating increased local inflammation. This stimulation accelerates the body's natural response to soft tissue repair by causing a "cascade effect," in which it increases the amount of blood, nutrients, and fibroblasts to the area. Furthermore, this results in the synthesis of collagen and eventual maturation of the tissue.

One method of action is influencing the tissue quality of the fascia. Fascia bundles surround the muscles allowing them to move upon each other and prevent muscle fibers from adhering to other. Over time and with age, the fibers can adjoin between layers of fascia causing stiffness, which creates faulty movement patterns due to this decreased range of motion (ROM). IASTM serves to restore optimal fascia quality resulting in less stiffness, increased ROM, and improved function. IASTM also affects other tissue types, such as collagen. Molecular cross-links within collagenous tissues also create adhesions and disrupt the normal tissue quality. Adhesions within the soft tissue which may have developed as a result of surgery, immobilization, repeated strain or other mechanisms, are broken down allowing full functional restoration to occur.

IASTM PHYSIOLOGY AND BENEFITS

Mechanical Effects

Studies have addressed the benefits of IASTM at the cellular level. Benefits include increased fibroblast proliferation, reduction in scar tissue, increased vascular response, and the remodeling of unorganized collagen fiber matrix following IASTM application.

Fibroblast is considered the most important cell in the extracellular matrix (ECM). The repair, regeneration and maintenance of soft tissue take place in the ECM. The fibroblast synthesizes the ECM, which includes collagen, elastin and proteoglycans, among many other essential substances. Fibroblasts have the ability to react as mechanotransducers, which means they are able to detect biophysical strain (deformation) such as compression, torque, shear and fluid flow, and create a mechanochemical response.

Neurophysiological Effects

Recent research has indicated that most forms of manual therapy has a neural mechanism in its effect. It initiates physiological actions that can cause changes in soft tissue like tone, plasticity and fluid dynamics.

In the case of IASTM, we are influencing the skin and the fascia beneath it. The skin and fascia are highly innervated with sensory nerve fibers, and the fascia has been found to contain up to 10 times as many mechanoreceptors as muscle tissue. These mechanoreceptors are stimulated which influences the central nervous system and the autonomic nervous system to cause a tonus change in the fascial structure. So a slow stroking using IASTM over the skin and underlying fascia influences the muscles below it causing inhibition of the Gamma motor system, causing a decrease in muscle tone. The stimulation of the mechanoreceptors also causes a reflex response that lowers overall muscle tonus and induces a whole body relaxation as well as an effect on the local area.

Clinical Benefits

The clinical benefits of IASTM are improvements in range of motion, strength and pain perception following treatment.

Overall, the expected outcome of IASTM is the stimulation of tissue repair, leading to decreased pain and stiffness, increased range of motion and function, and decreased total treatment time.

Benefit to the Clinician

IASTM provide clinicians with a mechanical advantage, thus preventing over-use to the hands. A study surveying physical therapists, found that after spinal pain, the second most common cause for absenteeism from work was overuse of the thumb. Ninety-one percent of physiotherapists using some sort of massage had to modify their treatment techniques because of thumb pain.

GENERAL BENEFITS OF IASTM

- Reduces overall treatment time and speeds up recovery of the patient
- Reduces the dependency on anti-inflammatory medicines, which can have side effects on the body
- Permanent resolution of chronic conditions.

INDICATIONS

- Limited motion
- Pain during motion
- Motor control issues
- Muscle recruitment issues

COMMON CONDITIONS FOR WHICH IASTM IS USED

- Medial epicondylitis, lateral epicondylitis
- Carpal tunnel syndrome
- Neck pain
- Plantar fasciitis
- Rotator cuff tendinitis
- Patellar tendinitis
- Tibialis posterior tendinitis
- Heel pain/Achilles tendinitis
- DeQuervain's syndrome
- Post-surgical and traumatic scars
- Myofascial pain and restrictions

- Musculoskeletal imbalances
- Chronic joint swelling associated with sprains/strains
- Ligament sprains
- Muscle strains
- Non-acute bursitis
- Reflex sympathetic dystrophy (RSD)
- Back pain
- Trigger finger
- Hip pain (replacements)
- It band syndrome
- Shin splints
- Chronic ankle sprains
- Acute ankle sprains (advanced technique)
- Scars (surgical, traumatic).

CONTRAINDICATIONS
- Deep vein thrombosis
- Kidney infections
- Rheumatoid arthritis
- Uncontrolled hypertension
- Osteomyelitis
- Osteoporosis
- Generalized infection
- Fractures
- Compromised tissue integrity (open wound, infection, tumor)
- Unhealed suture site/sutures
- Thrombophlebitis
- Patient intolerance/non-compliance
- Hypersensitivity
- Hematoma
- Myositis ossificans.

PRECAUTIONS FOR USE
- Varicose veins
- Neoplastic disorders/cancer
- Burn scars
- Acute inflammatory conditions (i.E. Synovitis)
- Pregnancy
- Anticoagulant medication

- Extra care should be taken for clean up in individuals with blood-borne diseases (HIV/AIDS).

TECHNIQUES
General Guidelines
- The tool should be applied at a 30–60° angle for a comfortable and good result.
- Treatment can be delivered in single directions or multiple directions as if you were treating a spider web under the instrument or your hand.
- Treatment should proceed from superior to inferior, inferior to superior, medial to lateral, lateral to medial and diagonally in all directions.
- The treatment should be administered for 30 seconds to 1–2 minutes before reassessing, then adding additional 30 second to 1-minute treatments in multiple directions as required.
- In order to avoid bruising and painful treatment, when using the tool, follow the procedure below:
  - Some patients are known to bruise easily so **please ask your patient prior to treatment** if they bruise early and if they do, reduce the amount of treatment pressure applied.
  - Use a 0-10 pain rating scale. Explain to the patient that treatment should range between 0 and 5 in the scale. Level 5 means the pain is tolerable but please do not add additional pressure. Remember also that every patient's Level 5 will differ.
  - Patient should be informed that they might sustain bruising, petechia (small red dots, or a mild scrape looking lesion), some soreness or mild pain or discomfort.
  - Always clean and sterilize the instruments after each patient. A Cavicide, Clorox, various hand wipes and other cleaners should be considered.
  - Use an emollient to reduce friction between the instrument and skin.

TYPES OF STROKE
Scan Stroke (Fig. 15.4)
- The stroke is used to run the instrument over the tissue in an attempt to detect a different feel from one area to another.

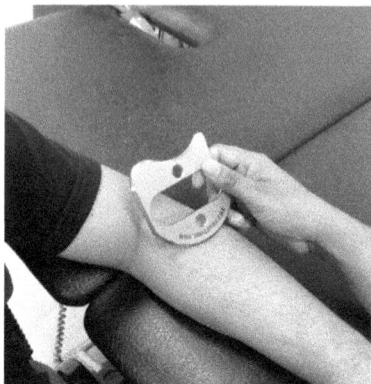

Fig. 15.4: Scan stroke.

- This is used to detect irregularities under the skin such as adhesions and increased tone
- Stroke is applied from superior to inferior, medial to lateral and diagonally to detect irregularities.

Sweep Stroke

- Once the soft tissue consistency is determined, the sweep stroke is used as treatment.
- It is similar to scan stroke but it is applied depending on what treatment effects needed
  - Fast stroke: To breakdown adhesion and scar tissue
  - Slow stroke: To reduce tone.

Brush Stroke

- This is done by simply applying the sweep stroke with very little pressure (**very light force**) in a rapid movement.
- This is used to create and anesthetic effect or diminish the tickle issue.

IASTM should not be used as a sole method of treatment: As in any manual therapy treatment, supplementation with exercises and additional modalities, e.g. joint mobilization designed to correct biomechanical deficiencies by addressing musculoskeletal strength and muscle imbalances throughout the entire kinetic chain should be used in conjunction with IASTM.

16

Stretching Techniques

Krishna N Sharma

Stretching is a general terms that describe any therapeutic maneuver that increases the extensibility of restricted soft tissues.

APPLICATION
Indications
- Contractures
- Muscle shortening due to antagonist weakness
- Scar tissue formation
- Soft tissue adhesions
- Before starting fitness exercises to prevent musculoskeletal injuries
- Before starting vigorous exercise to minimize postexercise muscle soreness.

Contraindications
- Acute inflammation
- Acute injury of the tissue
- Hard end feel
- Hematoma
- Hypermobility of the joint
- Infection
- Non-union or delayed union fracture
- Sharp, acute pain with joint movement or muscle elongation
- Unhealed fracture.

TYPES OF STRETCHING
I would like to classify the stretching techniques as follows:
- ***Stretching of muscle***
  - Static stretching

- Active stretching
- Passive stretching
  - Dynamic stretching
  - Ballistic stretching
  - Proprioceptive neuromuscular facilitation (PNF) stretching
    - Hold relax (HR) or contract relax (CR)
    - Agonist contraction (AC)
    - Hold relax with agonist contraction (HR-AC)
  - Muscle energy techniques (MET)
- **Stretching of myofascia**
  - Myofascial release (MFR)
- **Stretching of peri-articular tissues**
  - Joint mobilization
- **Stretching of peripheral nerve**
  - Neural tissue mobilization
- **Stretching of other soft tissues**
  - Soft tissue manipulation.

Static Stretching

It is the most commonly used stretching technique. In this technique the muscle is taken to its first tissue stop and the position is held for 30 seconds. This process is repeated 5–10 times.

In *active static stretching*, the position is held by the muscle contraction. The patient moves the joint through its ROM and holds the stretched position just without any support. In *passive static stretching*, the movement is done by the therapist and the position is held with the support of any object or by manually by therapist.

According to *Professor Erik Witvrouw* of the Ghent University, the static stretching mainly affects the muscle tissues (whereas the ballistic stretching affects the tendons).

Dynamic Stretching

It is usually done before sports like sprinting and martial arts. In this technique, the muscles are stretched by the use of continuous movement patterns which looks like the exercise or sport to be performed. The purpose of dynamic stretching is to improve flexibility for a given sport or activity.

Ballistic Stretching

Ballistic stretching is the repeated bouncing type of stretching which is used for athletic drills to stretch the targeted muscle group. The client takes the muscle near to its limit and then bounces to stretch it further. The therapists usually do not recommend it to the patients due to the injury possibilities.

According to *Professor Erik Witvrouw* of the Ghent University, the ballistic stretching mainly affects the tendons (whereas the static stretching affects the muscle tissues). So the ballistic stretching may be useful after tenotomy or tendon transfer surgeries where the postoperative fibrosis reduce the muscle length.

Proprioceptive Neuromuscular Facilitation (PNF) Stretching

PNF stretching is a set of stretching techniques which uses autogenic Inhibition and reciprocal inhibition for inhibition of the target muscle.

Hold Relax (HR) or Contract Relax (CR)

In the term of stretching, the HR and CR is used interchangeably. In this technique, the target muscle is kept in stretched position and then the patient does an isometric contraction of the target muscle for 3-10 seconds followed by relaxation. The limb is then passively repositioned to the new increased range. After 3-10 seconds, the patient relaxes the muscle and then contract the antagonist to move the limb into a greater position of stretch.

Agonist Contraction (AC)

Here the agonist actually means the muscle opposite to the target muscle. In this technique, the patient concentrically contracts the muscle opposite to the range limiting muscle and holds the end range position for few seconds. After a brief period of rest, the patient repeats the same procedure.

Hold Relax with Agonist Contraction (HR-AC)

It is the combination of upper two techniques. It is performed by passive stretch of target muscle, followed by maximum isometric contraction of target muscle and passive stretch of target muscle again. After that, maximum concentric contraction of antagonist muscle is performed.

Muscle Energy Techniques

Muscle energy techniques use the concepts of *autogenic inhibition, reciprocal inhibition,* and *oculocervical reflex* to relax and then stretch the target muscle. The patient is asked to do isometric/concentric/eccentric contraction in a precisely controlled direction and intensity against a counterforce applied by the therapist.

Myofascial Release

Myofascial release techniques focus on relaxing the fascia by applying direct pressure on the body and using slow and sometimes deep pressure to restore the extensibility of the fascia.

Joint Mobilization/Manipulation

These are the special manual therapy techniques specifically applied to joint structures to increase the extensibility of the periarticular structures to increase the ROM.

Neural Tissue Mobilization

The neural tissues are stretched and mobilized in the cases of adhesion or scar tissue around the nerve root or at the site of injury at the plexus or peripheral nerves after trauma or surgical procedures. Tension placed on the adhesions or scar tissue leads to pain or neurological symptoms.

Soft Tissue Manipulation

The soft tissue mobilization techniques involve various forms of deep massage and are used to increase the mobility of adherent or shortened connective tissues.

CHAPTER 17

Muscle Energy Technique

Krishna N Sharma

DEFINITIONS

It is a form of osteopathic manipulative diagnosis and treatment in which the patient's muscles are actively used on request, from a precisely controlled position, in a specific direction, and against a distinctly executed physician counterforce.
—**Education Council on Osteopathic Principles (ECOP)**

Muscle energy techniques are a class of soft tissue osteopathic (originally) manipulation methods that incorporate precisely directed and controlled, patient initiated, isometric and/or isotonic contractions, designed to improve musculoskeletal function and reduce pain.
—**Leon Chaitow**

In the above statement by *Leon Chaitow*, I personally would like to change the term *isotonic* to *concentric/eccentric* as the isotonic contractions are practically impossible, because during any motion the tone keep changing according to the mechanical advantage/disadvantage achieved due to the constantly changing angle of pull.

HISTORY

The current form of muscle energy technique (MET) is not the developed by any single person, but it is developed by various osteopathy practitioners.

The first person who used muscle energy in the 1940's and 1950's was *Dr TJ Ruddy* (1961)—an osteopathic doctor. He used to use a series of rapid, low amplitude muscle contractions against resistance at a rate of almost 20 pulsation in 10 seconds. He called it *Ruddy's Rapid Resistive Duction,* which has become *Pulsed MET* now.

Later on in 1958, *Dr Fred Mitchell, Sr.* (Fig. 17.1) took the principles of Dr Ruddy's and another osteopathy physician Carl Kettler, and incorporated them in the Manual Medicine. Though he never wrote any book or paper specifically on MET, he is called the *Father of Muscle Energy Techniques* because of his remarkable contributions in developing and spreading the MET. From 1950 to 1970, many physicians came to Chattanooga to learn his techniques. Hopefully this motivated him to systematize his ideas. He taught the first of six Muscle Energy Tutorials from March 3-7, 1970, at Fort Dodge, Iowa, to a osteopathic physicians group. Later on these tutorials were taught at Colorado Springs, CO, Milwaukee, WI, Dallas, TX, and St. Petersburg, FL.

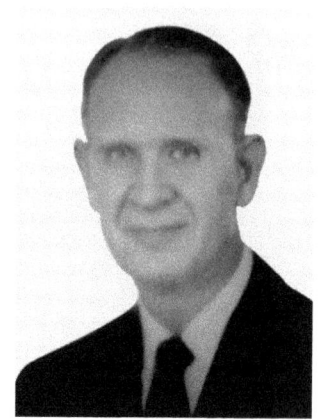

Fig. 17. 1: Dr Fred Mitchell Sr.

After his death in 1974, his son, *Dr Fred Mitchell, Jr.*, continued his work. He published the first text on MET—*An Evaluation and Treatment Manual of Osteopathic Manipulative Procedures* in 1973. It was based on the notes taken by one of his student PS Moran from his lecture at KCCOS. In 1973, Fred Mitchell, Jr. joined the faculty at College of Osteopathic Medicine at Michigan State University and after the death of his father in 1974, the Michigan State University offered the first CME course on MET principally taught by FL Mitchell, Jr. They developed it with time and they published the first textbook on MET with the same title—*An Evaluation and Treatment Manual of Osteopathic Manipulative Procedures* in 1979 which became out of print in 1991. And then finally they published a detailed book on MET—*The Muscle Energy Manual* in 3 volumes (in 1995, 1998, and 1999). In his book he defined it as when the patient uses his/her muscles on request, from a precisely controlled position in specific direction against distinctly executed counterforce.

In 1991, *Dr Sandra Yale* an osteopathic physician found the MET potentially beneficial in even severely ill and fragile patients. She said—*"The muscle energy techniques are particularly effective in patients who have severe pain from acute somatic dysfunction, such as those with a whiplash injury from a car accident, or a patient with severe muscle spasm from a fall. MET methods are also an excellent treatment modality for hospitalized or bedridden patients. They can be used in older patients who may have severely restricted motion from arthritis, or who have brittle osteoporotic bones."*

In 1996, a professor of biomechanics—*Dr Philip Greenman* summarized the potential benefits of the MET. He said *"The function of any articulation of the body, which can be moved by voluntary muscle action, either directly or indirectly, can be influenced by muscle energy procedures... Muscle energy techniques can be used to lengthen a shortened, contractured or spastic muscle; to strengthen a physiologically weakened muscle or group of muscles; to reduce localized edema, to relieve passive congestion, and to mobilize an articulation with restricted mobility."*

There were few other MET clinicians like *Edward Stiles, J Goodridge*, and *W Kuchera* who contributed a lot in developing the MET. Now the biggest name in the MET is *Dr Leon Chaitow* whose book—*Muscle Energy Techniques* (first issue published in 1996) is followed all over the world as the reference book for MET.

PHYSIOLOGY

The MET works in three ways.

Post-isometric Relaxation (PIR)

It is the reduction in the muscle tone just after a strong isometric contraction due to *autogenic inhibition*. Any strong contraction triggers the *Golgi tendon organ (GTO)* located in the tendon of agonist muscle. The impulse from the GTO meets with inhibitory motor neurons in the spinal cord after entering through the dorsal root. The inhibitory motor neurons stop the discharge of the efferent (motor) neuron's impulses and inhibit the further contraction of the agonists. It causes the decrease in the agonist muscle tone.

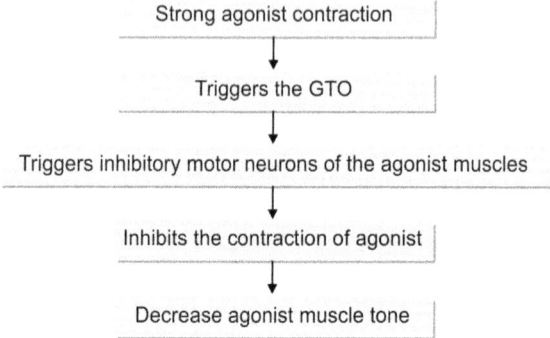

Reciprocal Inhibition (RI)

This is already known that if we activate the agonist muscle, the antagonist muscle is inhibited *(reciprocal inhibition)*. So even in the MET, the contraction of agonist muscles triggers the muscle spindles. The impulse from the spindles meets with inhibitory motor neurons of the antagonists in the spinal cord after entering through the dorsal root. The inhibitory motor neurons stop the discharge of the efferent (motor) neuron's impulses to the antagonists and inhibit the antagonists. It causes the decrease in the antagonist muscle tone.

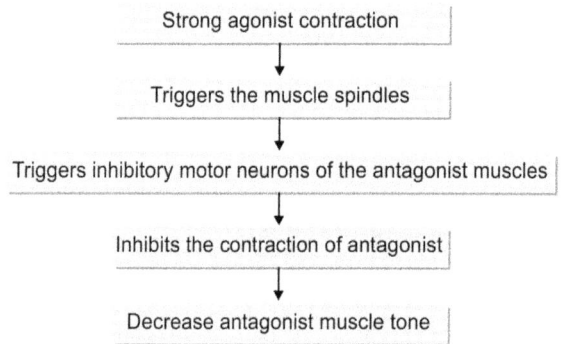

Oculocervical Reflex (OR)

The oculocervical reflex causes certain cervical and truncal muscles contraction on specific eye movements. It can be utilized to induce post-isometric relaxation effect or reciprocal inhibitory effect. It is very useful in the patients with severe neck or upper thoracic pain, strain, or spasm.

Muscle Energy Technique

APPLICATION
Indications
- Muscle contracture
- Spasticity
- Muscle weakness
- Malpositioning of a bony element
- Decreased joint ROM.

Contraindications
- Acute musculoskeletal injuries
- Unhealed fracture
- Joint instability
- Joint adhesion.

Precautions
- Unknown pathology
- Stress fracture
- Osteoporosis
- Tumors
- Strain
- Infection
- Diseases causing musculoskeletal pain.

General Considerations
The following steps must be followed for proper execution of the technique.
1. Positions the muscle, joint, or bone to be treated at the edge of the restrictive barrier in all three planes of motion and keep it slightly loose at one axis.
2. Instructs the patient to contract the muscle for 3–5 seconds in a particular direction against resistance.
3. Instruct the patient to completely relax the muscle.
4. Now slowly repositions the patient to the edge of the new restrictive barrier.
5. Repeat all the steps mentioned above for 3–7 times.
6. Reevaluate the patient to determine the effectiveness of the technique.

TECHNIQUES

Isometric Contraction (Utilizing Autogenic Inhibition)

The agonist muscle is kept close to the restriction barrier, and the patient does isometric contraction of the agonist for 3-4 seconds. Now the muscle is repositioned according to its new extended range. This process is repeated for 3-4 times.

Isometric Contraction (Utilizing Reciprocal Inhibition)

The antagonist muscle is kept close to the restriction barrier, and the patient does isometric contraction of the agonist for 3-4 seconds. Now the muscle is repositioned according to its new extended range. This process is repeated for 3-4 times.

Isotonic Concentric Contraction (Utilizing Autogenic Inhibition)

The agonist muscle is kept in resting length (comfortable mid-range) and the patient does concentric contraction of the agonist for 3-4 seconds against resistance. Now the muscle is repositioned according to its new extended range. This process is repeated for 3-4 times.

Isotonic Concentric Contraction (Utilizing Reciprocal Inhibition)

It is same as the above techniques, but instead of agonist, the patient contracts antagonist. It utilizes reciprocal inhibition.

Isotonic Eccentric Contraction

The muscle is kept close to the restriction barrier, and the patient does eccentric contraction of the agonist for 3-4 seconds. Now the muscle is repositioned according to its new extended range. This process is repeated for 3-4 times. It is better not to use this technique on head and neck muscles.

GUIDELINE

- Keep contractions light (20-30% of strength)
- Never over-stretch
- Take the patient's help to locate restriction barrier
- Patient should not experience any pain or discomfort.

CHAPTER 18

Myofascial Release

Krishna N Sharma

DEFINITION

"Myofascial release technique is a system of diagnosis and treatment first described by Andrew Taylor Still and his early students, which engages continual palpatory feedback to achieve release of myofascial tissues"

—**The Educational Council on Osteopathic Principles**

The myofascial release (MFR) is an umbrella term used to describe the approaches and techniques which are used to relieve the abnormal constriction of tense fascia. Fascia is the soft tissue component of the connective tissue which provides strength, support, elasticity, protection, and cushion to the body. It is made up of collagen, elastin, and polysaccharide gel complex. It can become restricted due to overuse, trauma, inactivity, or psychogenic disease, and may result in pain and muscle tension. The term myofascial was first used in medical literature by *Janet G Travell* in the 1940s in reference to musculoskeletal pain syndromes and trigger points. The myofascial release originated from the concept by *Andrew Taylor Still* in the late 19th century. According to *Robert Ward*, the term "myofascial release" as a technique was coined in 1981 when it was used as a course title at *Michigan State University*.

PHYSIOLOGICAL PRINCIPLES

According to *DiGiovanna and Schiowitz*, the physiological principles behind the effect of MFR are as follows:
- *Crossed extensor reflex:* The stretch reflex stimulates agonist and contralateral antagonist simultaneously.
- *Increased circulation:* It provides better nutrition and washes out the harmful metabolic waste products.

- *Increased temperature:* It increases the tissue extensibility.
- *Increased venous and lymphatic drainage:* It decreases edema and swelling.
- *Reciprocal inhibition:* It causes inhibition of the antagonist muscles.
- *Stretch reflex:* It increases the tone in loosened areas of hypotonic muscles.
- The stretch reflex is sustained by the muscle spindle reflex.
- Relaxation of the contracted muscle decreases the O_2 demand of the muscle, decreases pain, and increases ROM.

APPLICATION

Indications

- Adhesions and scar tissue
- Fibromyalgia
- Low back pain
- Myofascial pain syndrome
- Myofasciitis
- Neck pain
- Tendinosis
- Tenosynovitis.

Contraindications

- Acute inflammation
- Acute strain/sprain
- Aneurism
- Arterial dissection
- Cellulitis
- Client use of anticoagulant medications
- Deep vein thrombosis
- Fracture
- Hematoma
- Joint hypermobility
- Malignancy
- Osteoporosis
- Severe edema
- Skin hypersensitivity
- Varicose veins.

METHODS
The myofascial release methods can be classified as follows:
- Direct myofascial release
  - Active direct myofascial release
  - Passive direct myofascial release
- Indirect myofascial release
  - Active indirect myofascial release
  - Passive indirect myofascial release.

Direct Myofascial Release
The direct method or *fascial twist* or *deep tissue work* came from the osteopathy school in the 1920s by Neidner. In this method, the tissue is loaded with a constant force using knuckles, elbows, or other tools to slowly stretch the restricted fascia until release occurs. The therapist moves slowly through the layers of the fascia until the deep tissues are reached. The fascia is manipulated in opposition to the direction that the fascia may freely allow movement. Usually the direct-release techniques show immediate response.

According to *Michael Stanborough*, the direct myofascial release method is as follows:
- Land on the surface of the body with the appropriate 'tool' (knuckles, or forearm, etc.)
- Sink into the soft tissue
- Contact the first barrier/restricted layer
- Put in a 'line of tension'
- Engage the fascia by taking up the slack in the tissue
- Finally, move or drag the fascia across the surface while staying in touch with the underlying layers
- Exit gracefully.

The active direct myofascial release is administered by the patients themselves and the passive direct myofascial release is administered by the therapist.

Indirect Myofascial Release
This method is based on the concept of *inherent force* which is the natural tendency toward tissue homeostasis. In this method the fascia is 'unwind' by a gentle stretch with only a few grams of pressure. The dysfunctional tissues are guided along the direction

of least resistance until free movement is achieved. According to Barnes, the indirect myofascial release method is as follows:
- Lightly contact the fascia with relaxed hands
- Slowly stretch the fascia until reaching a barrier/restriction
- Maintain a light pressure to stretch the barrier for approximately 3–5 minutes
- Prior to release, the therapist will feel a therapeutic pulse (e.g. heat)
- As the barrier releases, the hand will feel the motion and softening of the tissue.
- The key is sustained pressure over time.

The active direct myofascial release is administered by the patients themselves and the passive direct myofascial release is administered by the therapist.

TECHNIQUES

General Techniques

General techniques are the techniques described above in the direct and indirect techniques.

Skin Rolling

This technique is used to break the adhesion between the skin and layer of fascia, and between the superficial and deep layers of fascia. In this technique, the therapist holds a roll of skin and subcutaneous fascia between the fingers and thumbs and rolls it while lifting away from the body (Fig. 18.1).

Separation of Compartments

In this technique, the therapist tries to separate the muscular or fascial compartments. The therapist applies pressure with fingers or knuckles and moves up the border of the muscle or fascial compartment visualizing gently separating the compartments apart (Fig. 18.2).

Lifting or Rolling Muscle Compartments

In this technique, the muscle is slowly lifted away from the bone and then it is rolled until resistance is felt. This position is held in this position until the muscle slowly release in the direction of roll (Fig. 18.3).

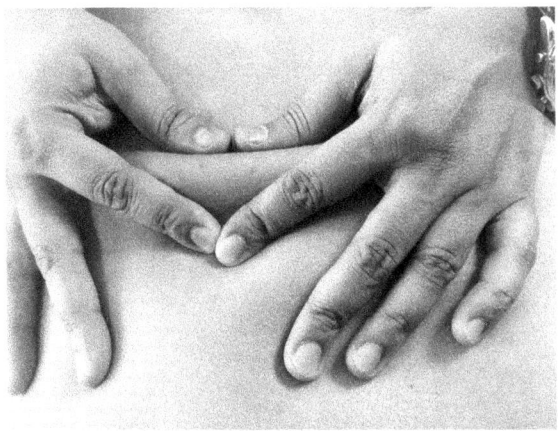

Fig. 18.1: Skin rolling.

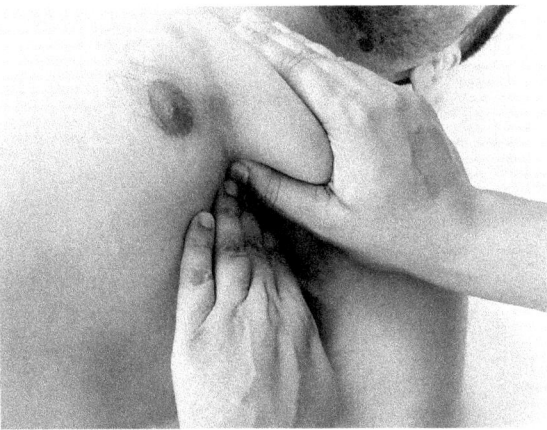

Fig. 18.2: Separation of compartments.

Placing Muscles into Stretched Position

In this technique, the therapist places the muscle in a relaxed stretch position which means that the stretch should not be enough to elicit stretch reflex. The gravity assisted position is preferred (Fig. 18.4).

Anchor and Stretch Strokes

In this technique, the therapist puts the muscle in relaxed position by flexing the joint and anchors on the area that is fibrotic/adhered/

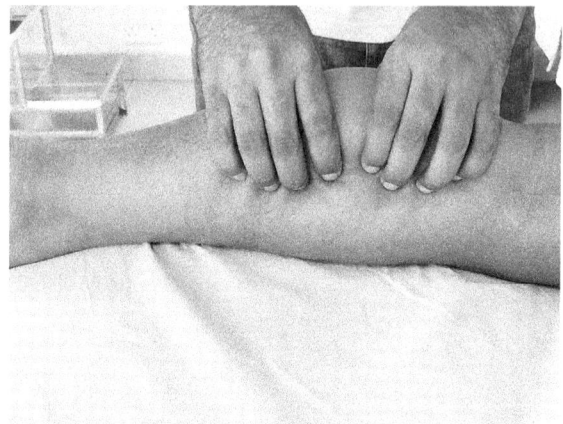

Fig. 18.3: Lifting or rolling muscle compartments.

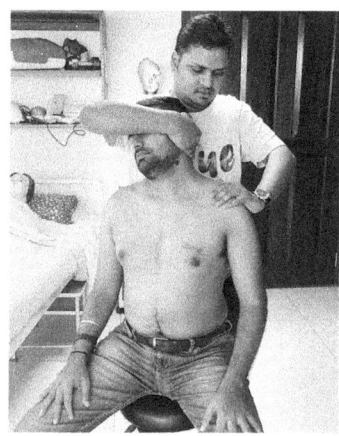

Fig. 18.4: Placing muscles into stretched position.

thickened with the precise tools, e.g. knuckles/fingers. After that he extends the joint so that the stretch is focused at that particular point of anchor. It is important that no sliding should take place below the anchored area so that the stretch may concentrate there (Fig. 18.5).

Expedited Lengthening Strokes

In this technique, the therapist puts the muscle in relaxed position by flexing the joint and then applies compression with movement of

Myofascial Release

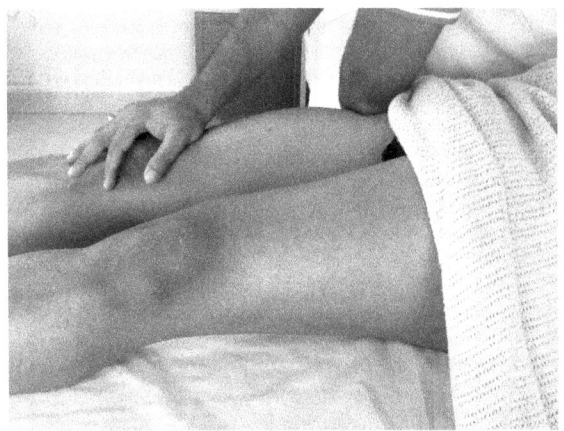

Fig. 18.5: Anchor and stretch strokes.

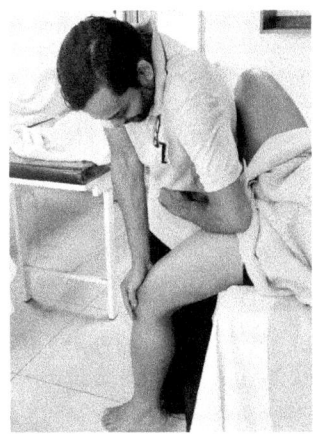

Fig. 18.6: Expedited lengthening strokes.

the myofascial compartment in the most expedient direction for the joint. It can be taken one step ahead by moving the joint to stretch fascia (Fig. 18.6).

CHAPTER

19 Trigger Point Release

Amit M Patel

TRIGGER POINT DEFINITIONS

A Trigger Point (TrPs) is a hyperirritable spot associated within a taut band of a skeletal muscle that is painful on compression or muscle contraction, and usually responds with a referred pain pattern distant from the spot. Very often there are nodules palpable within the muscle often at the size of 2-10 mm.
—Fernández-de-las-Peñas, C et al.

Trigger points are discrete, focal, hyperirritable spots located in a taut band of skeletal muscle. They produce pain locally and in a referred pattern and often accompany chronic musculoskeletal disorders.
—David J Alvarez, DO, and Pamela G Rockwell, DO, University of Michigan

In addition the author also wants to add that acute trauma or repetitive microtrauma may lead to the development of stress on muscle fibers and the formation of trigger points. Patients may have regional, persistent pain resulting in a decreased range of motion (ROM) in the affected muscles. These include muscles used to maintain body posture, such as those in the neck, shoulders, and pelvic girdle. Trigger points may also manifest as tension headache, tinnitus, temporomandibular joint pain, decreased range of motion in the legs, and low back pain.

HISTORY

Trigger point release, or similar theories has been around since the 19th century, however, there is no documentation that suggests the exact origin of trigger point release. Dating back to the 1940's the term myofascial was used in Janet Travell's research of different pain syndromes. In the 1950's there were articles that were published that talked about trigger points and myofascial pain.

The actual term of myofascial release was not used until 1981. It was used in the title of a course on myofascial release at Michigan State University. Trigger point release or myofacial trigger point release is based on the concepts created by Andrew Taylor Still, the founder of Osteopathic Medicine, in the 19th century. The first form of trigger point release that was used by Still was the indirect method. This method involves the gentle stretching of the fascia, such as the cross-hand technique. The indirect method was growing at the Kansas City College of Osteopathy and Surgery. Dr George Andrew Laughlin and Dr Esther Smoot were very influential in the growth of this indirect method.

The direct trigger point release most likely came about in the 1920's. This technique has developed much more slowly than the indirect technique. Dr William Neider developed this technique that was named "fascial twist," which was more forceful then the gentle stretching of the indirect method. Many of his concepts are present in today's techniques of trigger point release.

To effectively use trigger point release, a thorough understanding of its techniques is necessary.

PHYSIOLOGY

Fascia is a connective tissue along with tendons, ligaments, bone, and muscle. Fascia is divided into three different layers. The first layer, which is the superficial fascia, consists of connective tissue and adipose tissue. It provides a path for nerves and blood supply. The second layer of fascia is called the potential space. This area can become inflamed, which shows that it can be injured or stretched with any type of injury. The final layer of fascia is the deep layer. This layer is a very dense connective tissue that covers all the muscles and organs of the body. This layer also divides the different muscles from each other. The function of this layer is to allow movement of the muscles over each other, can provide attachments of some muscles, and it fills the spaces between some muscles and organs.

At times the muscles that are beneath and surrounded by this fascia become large rather quickly. This can cause the fascia to be too small and tight around the muscle. This causes restrictions in Range of Motion of a particular muscle. One function of trigger point release is to help stretch the fascia to allow more motion of the muscle therefore increasing the range of motion of the body.

Restrictions in motion and the cause of pain can also occur as a result of a muscle strain. A muscle strain can lead to chronic issues and inflammation. This pain can be a result of myofascial pain syndrome. Treatment of this type of pain has no real plan like the treatment of an acute injury has. This pain begins in the fascia and the muscle. This causes restrictions in range of motion and causes pain. If this is untreated, myofascial trigger points can then develop.

There are a few different theories regarding the origin of myofascial trigger points. One of them is the thought that abnormal muscle spindles send signals that may cause a trigger point. Another theory deals with scar tissue formation, while a third one talks about nerve signals can cause a myofascial trigger point. All of these can be causes of trigger points, however, researchers are not exactly sure of the origin of the trigger points.

Different techniques of trigger point release can help work out these trigger points and decrease pain and restore motion. Adhesions and scar tissue build-up can also be a cause of decreased motion and increased pain. Myofascial release can be used to reduce these adhesions and restore motion and decrease the associated pain from the lack of function.

Physiology of Stretching

Static stretching is a technique very commonly used to help improve range of motion of a particular body part and help reduce the risk of injury. The principal behind static stretching is the stress-strain curve, which demonstrates the extensibility and breaking point of tissue. Muscle will stretch when a force is placed on it. When the muscle is stretched beyond its original length it will then stay at the new length if the force is great enough.

Continuous stretching over a long period of time will result the muscle to elongate and become more flexible. This will cause the range of motion to increase and therefore help reduce the risk of injury from a tensile force. If the muscle is more flexible, it obviously can stretch further. When a strong tensile force is placed on the muscle, it can go further than it originally could, making it harder for the muscle to tear.

APPLICATION
Indications
- Muscle contracture
- Back pain
- Neck pain
- Fibromyalgia
- Repetitive strain injuries
- Muscular imbalances, which lead to overuse in isolated joints and faulty movement patterns.

Contraindications
- Acute fractures and healing fractures
- Acute strain or sprain
- Dislocation
- Neurologic or vascular compromise
- Osteoporosis or osteopenia
- Skin conditions
- Areas with heavy edema
- Malignancy
- Aneurysm
- Acute rheumatoid arthritis
- Advanced diabetes
- Infection (e.g. osteomyelitis).

DIAGNOSIS

When examining the patient who has presented with acute or chronic enigmatic pain, the physiotherapist must first conduct a thorough, time-consuming history and physical examination to identify what conditions are contributing to the patient's pain and to determine whether there is a significant myofascial component. If it appears likely that the patient does have chronic myofascial pain syndrome, the diagnostic task becomes two fold. In addition to identifying which trigger points (TrPs) in which muscles, are causing what portion of the patient's total pain complaint, the examiner must determine what perpetuating factors converted the initial acute myofascial pain syndrome to a chronic one. Myofascial TrPs may be perpetuated by mechanical (structural or postural) factors, by systemic factors, by associated medical conditions, and by psychological stress.

The central nervous system powerfully modulates pain input from the muscles in ways that can explain referred pain and altered sensation from TrPs. In phase 1 (constant pain from severely active TrPs), patients may already have such intense pain that they do not perceive an increase and cannot distinguish what makes it worse. Phase 2 (pain from less irritable TrPs that is perceived only on movement and not at rest) is ideal for educating the patient as to which muscles and movements are responsible for the pain, and how to manage it. In phase 3 (latent TrPs that are causing no pain), the patient still has some residual dysfunction and is vulnerable to reactivation of the latent TrPs.

Trigger Points Physical Examination

Specific trigger points examination of the muscles is undertaken following a complete general physical examination. When searching for active TrPs that are responsible for the patient's pain, it is essential to know the precise location of the pain and to know which specific muscles can refer pain to that location. Muscles that could be causing the pain are tested for restriction of passive stretch range of motion and for pain at the shortened end of active range of motion, as compared with uninvolved contralateral muscles. Suspected muscles are also tested for mild-to-moderate weakness either by conventional isometric strength testing or during a lengthening contraction. Such weakness is not associated with atrophy of the muscle.

The muscles showing abnormalities in these tests are the ones most likely to have the taut bands and spot tenderness of the TrP. The taut bands are located by palpation and then tested for a local twitch response and reproduction of the patient's pain complaint by digital pressure on the TrP. One must try to distinguish active TrPs from latent ones, which can also respond positively to the tests described but are not responsible for a pain complaint. Active TrPs are more irritable than latent TrPs and show greater responses on examination. If inactivation of the suspected TrP does not relieve the pain, it may either have been a latent TrP or it may not have been the only active TrP referring pain to that area.

Examination for mechanical perpetuating factors requires careful observation of the patient's postures, body symmetry, and movement patterns. Common mechanical factors that can influence many muscles are the round-shouldered, head-forward posture with loss of normal lumbar lordosis, and body asymmetries including a lower limb-length inequality and a small hemipelvis. Tightness of the iliopsoas and hamstring muscles can also seriously disrupt balanced posture.

DIFFERENTIAL DIAGNOSIS

The most important differential diagnosis is tender points.

Tender Points

Tender points, common in fibromyalgia, are discrete areas of tenderness over muscle, bone, tendon, and fat that cause local pain and are tender to palpation. Patients do not jump when tender points are palpated. Tender points do not refer pain to nearby or distant locations. These two pain syndromes may overlap in symptoms and are difficult to differentiate without a thorough examination by a skilled physician. Although they may be concomitant and may interact with one another.

1. Non-myofascial tender points
2. Musculoskeletal diseases:
   - Temporomandibular joint disorders
   - Occupational myalgias
   - Post-traumatic hyperirritability syndrome
   - Joint dysfunction (osteoarthritis)
   - Tendonitis and bursitis
3. Neurological disorders:
   - Trigeminal neuralgia
   - Glossopharyngeal neuralgia
   - Sphenopalatine neuralgia
4. Systemic diseases
   - Rheumatoid arthritis
   - Gout
   - Psoriatic arthritis
   - Infections (viral, bacterial and/or protozoan)
5. Heterotopic pain of central origin
6. Axis II-type disorders
   - Psychogenic pain
   - Painful behaviors
   - Prug reactions.

TECHNIQUES

Direct Trigger Point Release

The direct trigger point release method engages the myofascial tissue "restrictive barrier" (tension). The tissue is loaded with a constant force until "release" occurs. Direct release is sometimes called "deep tissue work", a misnomer as some of the important tissues are quite superficial. Physiotherapist uses knuckles, elbows, or other tools to slowly stretch the fascia by applying a few kilograms—force or tens of Newtons. Direct trigger point release is an attempt to bring about changes in the myofascial structures by stretching or elongation of fascia, or mobilizing adhesive tissues. The physiotherapist moves slowly through the layers of the fascia until the deeper tissues are reached.

Direct trigger point release technique is applied as below:
- Land on the surface of the body with the appropriate 'tool' (knuckles, or forearm, etc.)
- Sink into the soft tissue
- Contact the first barrier/restricted layer
- Put in a 'line of tension'
- Engage the fascia by taking up the slack in the tissue
- Finally, move or drag the fascia across the surface while staying in touch with the underlying layers
- Exit gracefully.

Indirect Trigger Point Release

The indirect method involves a gentle stretch, with only a few grams of pressure, which is said to allow the fascia to "unwind" itself, guiding the dysfunctional tissue "along the path of least resistance until free movement is achieved."

Indirect trigger point release technique is applied as below:
- Lightly contact the fascia with relaxed hands
- Slowly stretch the fascia until reaching a barrier/restriction
- Maintain a light pressure to stretch the barrier for approximately 3-5 minutes
- Prior to release, the therapist will feel a therapeutic pulse (e.g. heat)
- As the barrier releases, the hand will feel the motion and softening of the tissue
- The key is sustained pressure over time.

GENERAL CONSIDERATIONS AND RULES

1. The physiotherapist palpates the patient using layer by layer palpatory principles and with just enough pressure to capture the skin and subcutaneous facial structures. Any movement of the hand on the skin should cause the skin to move along with the hand over the skin.
2. The physiotherapist gently moves the palpating hand or hands in the linear direction of choice (hands of the clock) moving through the x-axes and y-axes.
3. Symmetry versus the asymmetry of tissue compliance is noted in the linear directions tested.
4. The physiotherapist may add a variety of directions of motion, including other linear movements in a 360 degree reference and clockwise and counter-clockwise rotational manner.
5. The pressure that the physiotherapist uses to determine compliance may be minimal to moderate, depending on the clinical presentation of the patient (acute painful versus chronic minimally painful) and what the physiotherapist believes is appropriate for the situation.
6. After determining the ease and bind barriers of the tissue in these directions, the physiotherapist determines whether gentle or moderate pressures in a direct (towards bind) or indirect (towards ease) technique is appropriate.
7. The physiotherapist slowly moves the hand controlled myofascial tissues toward the appropriate barrier, and on meeting the barrier, he or she holds the tissue at that point without relieving the pressure. The physiotherapist should notice that after 20 to 30 seconds, a change of tissue—compliance occurs; this is demonstrated by movement of tissue through the originally determined barrier (creep or fascial creep).
8. The physiotherapist follows this change and continues holding until no further evidence of creep occurs. There may be a number of compliance changes (creep) before this phenomenon stops.
9. The physiotherapist reevaluates the tissue to determine whether the tissue's compliance and quality have improved. The technique may be repeated at the same area or another and follow-up visits may be prescribed for a 3-day interval or longer, depending on patient's reactivity.

AREAS OF TRIGGER POINT SYNDROMES

- Trapezius
- Sternocleidomastoideus
- Masseter
- Temporalis
- Pterygoideus medialis
- Pterygoideus lateralis
- Digasticus
- Orbicularis oculi
- Zygomaticus major
- Platysma
- Scalp
- Splenius
- Deep muscles of the neck
  - Semispinalis capitis
  - Semispinalis cervicis
  - Multifundi
- Upper muscles of the neck
  - Rectus capitis
  - Obliquus capitis
- Levator scapule
- Scalenus
- Supraspinatus
- Infraspinatus
- Teres minor
- Latissimus dorsi
- Teres major
- Subscapularis
- Rhomboideus
- Deltoideus
- Coracobrachialis
- Biceps brachii
- Brachialis
- Triceps brachii
- Anconeus
- Extensors carpi
  - Extensor carpi radialis longus
  - Extensor carpi radialis brevis
  - Extensor carpi ulnaris
  - Brachioradialis

- Extensor digitorum
- Supinator
- Palmaris longus
- Flexors carpi—digitorum
  - Flexor carpi radialis
  - Flexor carpi ulnaris
  - Flexor digitorum superficialis
  - Flexor digitorum profundus
  - Flexor policis longus
  - Pronator teres
- Opponens—adductor policis
- Interosseous
  - Interossei
  - Abductor digiti minimi
- Pectoralis major and subclavicularis
- Sternalis
- Serratus superior posterior
- Serratus anterior
- Serratus inferior posterior
- Paravertebralis
  - Iliocostalis
  - Semispinalis
  - Multifundi
  - Rotators
- Regio abdominalis
  - Obliquus abdominis
  - Transversus abdominis
  - Rectus abdominis
  - Pyramidalis
- Quadratus lumborum
- Iliopsoas
- Pelvic floor muscles
  - Bulbospongiosus
  - Ischiocavernosus
  - Transversus perinei
  - Sphincter ani
  - Levator ani
  - Coccygeus
  - Obturator internus

- Gluteus maximus
- Gluteus medius
- Gluteus minimus
- Short lateral rotators
  - Gemelli
  - Quadratus femoris
  - Obturator internus
  - Obturator externus
- Tensor fasciae latae sartorius
- Pectineus
- Quadriceps femoris group
  - Rectus femoris
  - Vastus medialis
  - Vastus intermedius
  - Vastus lateralis
- Adductor
  - Adductor longus
  - Adductor brevis
  - Adductor magnus
  - Gracilis
- Hamstring muscles
  - Biceps femoris
  - Semitendinosus
  - Semimembranosus
- Popliteus
- Tibialis anterior
- Peroneal muscles
  - Peroneus longus
  - Peroneus brevis
  - Peroneus tertius
- Gastrocnemius
- Soleus plantaris
- Tibialis posterior
- Long extensors of toes
  - Extensor digitorum longus
  - Extensor hallucis longus
- Long flexor muscles of toes
  - Flexor digitorum longus
  - Flexor hallucis longus

- Superficial intrinsic foot muscles
  - Extensor digitorum brevis
  - Extensor hallucis brevis
  - Abductor hallucis
  - Flexor digitorum brevis
  - Abductor digiti minimi
- Deep intrinsic foot muscles
  - Quadratus plantar
  - Lumbricals
  - Flexor hallucis brevis
  - Adductor hallucis
  - Flexor digiti minimi brevis
  - Interossei.

CHAPTER

20 Kinesiological Taping

Piyush Jain

Kinesiological taping is a rehabilitative-cum protective use of stretchable kinesiological tapes to provide reduction of pain, enhancing performance, preventing injuries, support to the joints, repositioning of structure as well and for fascial and ligamentous correction. It facilitate the healing process while providing full range of motion with support to the joint's supportive structures as well as mobilization effects. Kinesiological tapes are widely used in nearly all sports injuries, orthopedic conditions, neurological rehabilitation as well as gynecological and pediatric conditions.

The kinesiological tapes are being used from field games, hospitals, clinics and rehabilitation homes. Unlike standard athletic taping, which often involves wrapping a joint for support and compression, kinesiological tape is placed in a variety of patterns depending on the injury. It is pulled into differing degrees of tension to create the desired effect and is typically worn for 2–5 days, unlike standard tape, which is used mainly during an activity (Fig. 20.1).

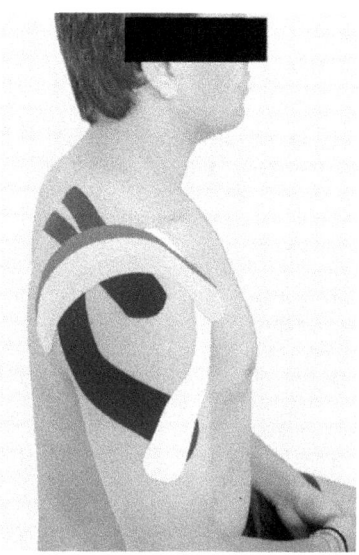

Fig. 20.1: Kinesiological tapes application for shoulder impingement syndrome.

Kinesiology taping is best used as an adjunct to physical therapy and exercise. It can unimaginably speeds up the rehabilitation process by lessening pain, providing support and correction and also improving tolerance to exercise and movement. The success of kinesiological taping strongly depends on therapist knowledge and skills. A thorough examination and use of clinical reasoning to find out the structure at fault is integral to determine which taping techniques are indicated. For instance, the clinician must know if the patient needs taping to assist muscle strengthening or to assist muscle relaxation, as the taping will be different. A good physiotherapy rehabilitation protocol goes hand-in-hand with proper taping and evaluation or assessment.

PROPERTIES OF KINESIOLOGICAL TAPES

Kinesiological tapes are made up of cotton, and contains small amount to no latex. The kinesiological tapes are 100% medication free and provide only physical effects not any medical effects so making it a non-side effective therapy. It has a light adhesive made from 100% acrylic, which is almost hypo-allergic (Fig. 20.2).

Kinesiological tapes comes in different sizes as 5 cm × 5 m, 2.5 cm × 5 m, 3.75 cm × 5 m, 7.5 cm × 5 m, but the commonly used tape size is 5 cm × 5 m which has approximately 8–15 applications depending on the structure and condition to be treated. Kinesiological tapes are available in various colors ranging from beige, blue, black, pink, red, orange, purple, etc. This color difference is only for the psychological factors like light colors are soothing and bright colors are aggressive and boosting. There are no effect on the quality and stretch ability of the tapes of different colors. They all possess the same properties and qualities.

Kinesiological tape stretches to approximately 140–150% of its original length. That means if we take a strip of 10 cm length, on stretching it can be maximally stretched up to 15 cm in total that is 10 cm original and 50% the total length. This concept have to be understood before starting taping technique, during application we use words like 10% stretch or 100% stretch which literally mean 10% of the

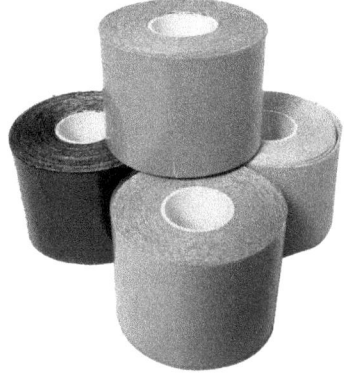

Fig. 20.2: Kinesiological tapes.

available stretch. That means if we say 10% stretch it will corresponds to only 5% of increase in original length. The kinesiological tapes come with 10% pre-stretched length. This pre-stretched length is always kept in mind while removing the backing paper as during application we can use this 10% stretch.

Kinesiological tapes consist of 100% acrylic which is a hypo-allergic substance, making it suitable for application to all the individuals. The acrylic glue is masked on the tape in a fixed sine wave pattern (Fig. 20.3). The cotton tape is woven such like that it can only be stretched in a particular longitudinal direction, and not in a transverse direction, this specific acrylic design helps in using the tape to increase or decrease the muscle tone as well as for functional correction. The energy stored in the tape on stretching is only used in one direction, which decreases the wasting of energy. When the tape is stretched it stores the potential energy, now due to its ability to stretch and recoil in longitudinal manner, all the potential energy is used in a specific direction, minimizing the energy loss as well as increasing the efficacy of the tapes.

Fig. 20.3: Kinesiological tape acrylic glue pattern.

The acrylic adhesive is heat activated. To activate the glue, rub the tape after application so as the therapist feels the warmth; this heat activates the glue and leads to proper adherence of tape onto the skin. It can be easily removed and leaves no sticky residue. Moisture dissipates quickly through the porous material of the tape. Due to its water resistant and hypo-allergic properties it can be worn from 2 to 5 days after application.

EFFECTS OF KINESIOLOGICAL TAPE

The kinesiological taping method is a therapeutic taping technique which not only offers the patient and player the support, but also the rehabilitation. By targeting different receptors within the somatosensory system, kinesiology tape alleviates pain and facilitates lymphatic drainage by microscopically lifting the skin. This lifting affect forms convolutions in the skin thus increasing

interstitial space and allowing for a decrease in inflammation of the affected areas. In short we may list the effects as:
- Stimulate or inhibit muscle function
- Enhances proprioception
- Support joints
- Fascial correction
- Pain relief
- Enhances lymphatic drainage.

Stimulate or Inhibit Muscle Function

Kinesiological tape's elastic properties can be used either to assist muscles during contraction, or inhibit their contraction. When the aim of application of tape is to provide or enhance muscle contraction, the tape base is applied without any stretch to the origin of the muscle, and then the muscle is taken into a stretched position and the tape is applied with no stretch or 10% stretch along the course of muscle. Due to recoil property and sine wave pattern of the glue and a fixed base, the tape will recoils toward the base, i.e. its origin, hence facilitating the muscle contraction.

When we need to get the inhibition of the muscle activity, we tape the muscle with the base at insertion with no stretch and then keeping the muscle in stretched position, tape is applied throughout the length of muscle till origin, this helps in relieving or inhibiting the muscle activity and is helpful in decreasing the tone and increasing the length of shortened muscles.

Enhances Proprioception

Kinesiology tape can be used to create pressure over ligaments and tendons to improve proprioception and dynamic stability. This also has been theorized to stimulate mechanoreceptors thus improving proprioception. Proprioception means 'sense of self'. In the limbs, the proprioceptors are sensors that provide information about joint angle, muscle length, and muscle tension, which is integrated to give information about the position of the limb in space. The muscle spindle is one type of proprioceptors that provides information about changes in muscle length. The Golgi tendon organ is another type of proprioceptors that provides information about changes in muscle tension. Thus when the tape is applied it sends the stimulus either by inhibiting or facilitating the muscle action to the brain and help in enhanced proprioception.

Support Joints

Kinesiological taping is very useful in supporting and protecting the joint while providing complete range of motion. The supporting structure of a joint such as ligament can be taped with ligamentous taping technique so as to provide more stability and support to the ligaments and joint hence preventing injury. The individual ligament can be taped or the group of the ligaments (knee) can also be taped in a circumferential method so as to get joint stability.

Fascial Correction

Fascia is an intricate web of connective tissue that envelops the entire body underneath the skin, connecting muscles, bones, vessels, organs and more. When fascia becomes dysfunctional or tight, it affects the entire body and can cause altered movement patterns which can lead to injury or further dysfunction. The fascia is divided in three major layers—the superficial fascia (directly beneath the skin), the deep fascia (surrounding the muscles), and the subserous fascia (supporting the internal organs). The fascia surrounds muscles, groups of muscles, blood vessels, and nerves, binding some structures together, while permitting others to slide smoothly over each other. When there is any pathology between the fascia and the structure like muscle, there are formation of adhesion between the fascia and muscle, which will restrict the normal function of the muscle. The elastic properties of the kinesiological tapes can be used as myofascial release as well as it can last the effect, as it has an application time of 2-5 days. While application, the therapist fixes the base and applies a passive stretch or rhythmical correction to fascia and tape the structure with about 80-100% stretch. It not only helps in myofascial release but the effects are prolonged.

Pain Relief

Kinesiology tape is commonly applied to injured or painful muscles while the muscle is in stretched position, when the muscle or tissue is returned to its resting length after tape is applied, wrinkles are created in the taped area because of the elastic property of the tape and the potential energy stored in the tape. These wrinkles are the indication of lifting of the skin. This result in creating a space beneath the skin causing more area for blood and lymph to flow which in result relieves the pain by washing away the waste as well promotes healing. The tape also acts on the mechanoreceptors of the skin causing the relief in pain via the pain gate mechanism.

Enhancing Lymphatic Drainage

The kinesiological tape application for lymphatic drainage is a fan-shaped tape specially designed to reduce swelling, bruising and pain. Its unique fan-shaped design allows it to be positioned directly over the lymphatic channels responsible for removing excess fluids from the body. The tape exerts a lifting action on the skin, allowing fluid to drain more effectively. As the swelling recedes, this reduces irritation to pain receptors under the skin, leading to relief of pain in severely swollen areas.

Application

Kinesiological taping is used as therapeutic-cum rehabilitative modality in physiotherapy protocols. Prior to application of any of the therapeutic modality the prerequisite is proper evaluation of the patient or the subject. Merely naming a disease is not the evaluation, the use of clinical reasoning in evaluating helps to determine the structure at fault, which is the basic for accepting the type of tape pattern used. In the conventional taping method via stretchable tape using its complete stretch, the main aim was to limit the range of motion, function of joint or for protection from injury or re-injury. But using the concept of kinesiological taping is entirely different as it enhances or inhibit the muscle, support a structure and it allows protection in full range of motion.

CLINICAL COMPARISONS (TABLE 20.1)

Table 20.1: Clinical comparisons of kinesiological taping.

Clinical condition	Conventional taping	Kinesiology taping
Muscle weakness	Holds	Improves via elastic input
Pain	No effect on nociceptors	Stimulates analgesics in the skin
Muscle spasm	Unloads/holds	Relieves
Edema	May restrict fluid flow	Assists fluid flow
Range of motion	Limits motion	Enhances motion
Joint mechanics	Immobilizes	Gives input to joint receptors
Length of wear	1–2 days	Several days

PREPARATION OF PATIENT

The skin should be washed and properly dried. The skin should be free of oils and lotions, oil or dirt will limit the acrylic adhesives ability to adhere to the skin, and also limit both effectiveness and duration of application. For some subjects body hair may limit adhesion. If the body hair limits adhesion then the therapist needs to shave the area to be treated. In the area where there is moisture and more perspiration, a water resistant solution, or gel is pre-applied. This will limit the moisture and help in proper adhesion of the tape.

POSITION OF THE PATIENT

The patient should be comfortably positioned in such a way that the part on which taping is to done is freely movable. For example, for the application of tape on a deltoid, patient must be seated on a stool, or a couch in a high sitting position so as he/she can perform movement in full range. Similarly in case of ankle, patient can be allowed to lies on the couch with foot and ankle out of the couch and even the long sitting position can be used.

POSITION OF THE THERAPIST

The position of the therapist depends on the part to be treated and the course of tape to be applied. The therapist should adopt such a position from where he can cover the course of muscle, ligament or the structure to be taped. For example, for tape application to the trapezius upper fibers, the therapist can stand in front or back of the patient, similarly in case of application of tape to sciatic nerve course therapist usually stand in front of patient while the patient is in side-lying position and therapist hold the extremity.

KINESIOLOGICAL TAPE STRIPS

Types of strips commonly used in kinesiological taping:
- I strip
- Y strip
- X strip
- I strip with hole
- X strip with hole
- Fan shaped.

"I" shaped strips are commonly used strip during kinesiological taping, I strip is the required length of the tape, with its end rounded off. I strips are used for muscle application, ligament techniques and space correction techniques.

"Y" strip is a modified I strip which has a single base but is cut into two vertical strips from either end. The length of vertical cut depends on the length of muscle belly, e.g. taping for extensor pollicis longus, the muscle has a short belly and a long tendons end, the I strip is cut into the Y till the length of muscle belly and the tendinous part is taped with base or single strip. Y strips are used for muscle as well as for fascial correction and mechanical correction techniques.

"X" strips are modified Y strip, which has a single center and bifurcated from the both ends. X strips also called as double Y shaped. It is used in the areas where there are two joint muscle applications and the level of stretch differs with the course of the muscle.

I and X strips with hole at center are modification of these strip where there is a triangular hole in the middle of the strips, these are used in taping of area with bony prominence so as there is no restriction of the movement, for example, as in taping for olecranon bursitis, I strip and X are used at posterior aspect of elbow, so as to facilitate the extension, we cut a hole in center so as there is no restriction to olecranon movement.

Fan-shaped strips has a single based on one side, the other side its spilled or cut into 4 or 6 strips making it look like a hand fan, or multiple Y strips. These are used specifically for lymphatic application. It helps in activation of lymphatic ducts, improving circulation by creating space beneath the skin.

Pictures of Tapes (Figs. 20.4 to 20.7)

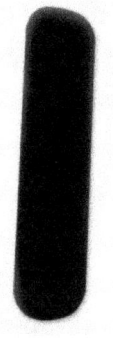

Fig. 20.4: I strip.

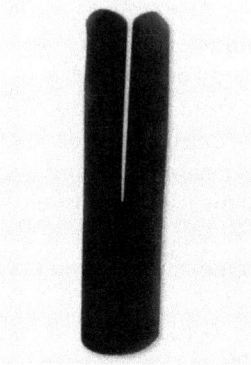

Fig. 20.5: Y strip.

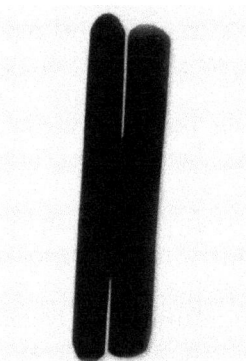

Fig. 20.6: X strip.

Fig. 20.7: Fan strip.

Kinesiological Taping

REMOVAL OF BACKING PAPER

The removal of tape from the backing paper is one of the most important part for proper application of the tape. The therapist must take every possible precaution to avoid touching the adhesive side of the tape.

There are two ways to remove the backing paper which depends on the type of application being used:

Application of Base

The therapist must hold the tape strip, vertically and by the use of the index finger just strip of the edge of backing paper so as just a corner is exposed, now the tape is removed so that the part that of the base is exposed from the paper, the backing paper is folded back prior to application of base, and then the base is fixed on the part to be treated. This removal technique is used in muscle application.

Application of Center

This technique is mainly used in ligament correction, or in space taping procedures where we need to apply the middle part first then the base. The therapist holds the strip horizontally with both hands, tearing the center of tape with paper, this result in tearing the backing paper not the tape, the backing paper is folded back and the tape is applied with even stretch to the part.

Picture of Removing of Backing Paper (Figs. 20.8 and 20.9)

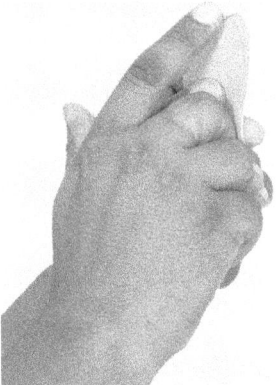

Fig. 20.8: Removal of backing paper.

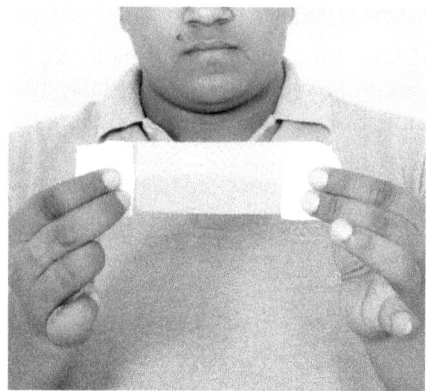

Fig. 20.9: Tearing of backing paper from center.

Four Taping Techniques 4TT's:
- Muscle taping technique (MTT).
- Ligament taping technique (LTT).
- Fascia correction taping technique (FCTT).
- Lymphatic corrective taping technique (LCTT).

Taping techniques has been classified into four basic group depending on the structure and outcome for which taping is to be done.

Muscle Taping Technique (MTT)

These taping techniques as understood by name, and are used to tape the muscular structures. In muscle taping, two techniques are used depending on the desired outcome: tonus up and tonus down technique.

Ligament Taping Technique (LTT)

Ligament taping is used to reinforce the ligamentous structure, with all the stretch maintained at center of tape. Ligament technique is also used as tendon technique and space technique.

Space Taping Techniques (STT)

This technique is used in the acute injury condition, pain areas and for trigger points. The method principle of STT is to use the recoil property of the tape to create space beneath the skin so as to promote flow of fluids and reducing pain by decreasing pressure as well.

Fascia Correction Taping Technique (FCTT)
This technique works on the biomechanical alignment of the structures like fascia and bones. This technique is used to correct a functional abnormality. FCTT is used as a corrective technique or a repositioning technique where aim is to realign or correct a biomechanical function of a bone like patella or for corrective alignment of vertebrae or for correction of fascial abnormality.

Lymphatic Correction Taping Technique (LCTT)
The LCTT is used to correct and increase the flow of lymph towards the lymphatic ducts so as to reduce the lymphedema and lymph statis. The fan-shaped strips are applied which stimulates the ducts and the recoiling effect of the strips create space and enhance lymph flow.

CHAPTER 21

Pilates

Tanvi Patole

Joseph Humbertus Pilates (Fig. 21.1) was born in 1880 in Germany. He was suffering from asthma, rheumatic fever and suspected of having tuberculosis in childhood. He worked very hard and improved his physical condition by the age of fourteen so that he was posing for anatomy chart. He developed skills in gymnastics, skiing and diving in his teenage life. He studied the musculature of the human body. He merged Eastern forms of exercise with his Westernstudies of physiology and movement, which was later known as Pilates method. This exercise program emphasizes on good posture, strength and flexibility of the body and also enhances awareness of body to support efficient and graceful movement. Also greater importance is given to the techniques in which they are performed than the number of repetitions.

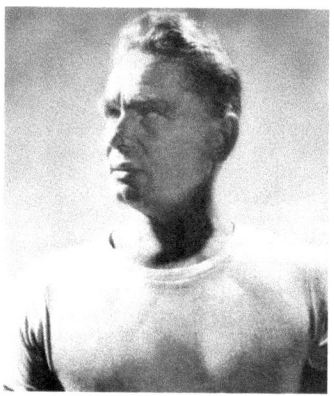

Fig. 21.1: Joseph Humbertus Pilates.

Pilates exercises help to stabilize the center or the 'Powerhouse' by activation of local stabilizers, inhibition of global musculature and proper breathing techniques. It helps to improve quality of movement which helps to improve quality of life. And it will also improve mental and physical conditioning.

PRINCIPLES

Alignment

Alignment or good posture is very important to practice Pilates. Head, shoulder girdle, rib cage and pelvis should be aligned in the correct or neutral position with respect to each other and maintain that position while performing exercises in Pilates. Awareness of the body parts is required to achieve the best out of each exercise and it also helps to prevent injury.

Concentration

Benefits of exercises are lost if movements are performed improperly. If exercises are performed with full commitment and attention, maximum value can be obtained from each movement you perform. Pilates demands intense focus.

Concentration is the most important and the first step in the learning process. Our initial movements may be jerky and awkward as our body tries to resist what our mind wants to perform. But when we focus and practice, we realize that even simple movements are difficult or complex to perform. Positions and movements of the body are interconnected. If the alignment is not proper, movement may get affected. As the level of precision in your movement improves, the quality of movement improves, which becomes noticeable.

Centering

Pilates brings the focus to the center of the body which the area between lower ribs and pubic bone which includes lower back, abdomen, buttocks and hips—the 'Powerhouse'. When the movements are performed, the powerhouse acts as a center of energy and it flows towards periphery. When the movements are performed the force and effort comes from the center. So the center is the most important to maintain a good control.

Breathing

Joseph Pilates emphasized on correct breathing pattern which helps in circulating the blood and carry nutrients to different parts of the body and carry away the wastes related to fatigue. It also improves stamina. If you are not breathing properly during exercises, gas exchange will not occur and as we know for the blood to do its work, it has to be charged with oxygen. So complete inhalation and exhalation is a part of this exercises. He wrote that breathing is the most integral part and even if one follows no other recommendation, learning to breathe correctly is the most important thing.

Control

Pilates exercise is done with complete muscular control. Alignment, concentration, effort and awareness of body position are important to perform movement. With the proper control you can regulate execution of movement. To achieve this refined control, you need lot of practice which will help in the development of strength and flexibility. This helps in the refinement of motor programs. When you learn to gain to control a movement, performance may get compromised. But as you learn, practice and achieve perfection in your movement, the greater control allows you to perform that same movement more quickly and with better performance.

Precision

Precision or exactness of exercise involves properly executed movement with great focus and understanding. Proper alignment of the body part and controlling movement at subconscious level helps to achieve graceful and fine tuning of the movement.

Flowing Movement

Smoothness and efficiency of movement should be performed through the use of appropriate transitions. When precision has been achieved, fluidity of movement is achieved while exercising. And when movements are in flow, muscles get toned.

BENEFITS OF PILATES

- Improves flexibility
- Enhances fitness level
- Increases muscle strength
- Enhances muscle control
- Improves performance
- Teaches you to move gracefully
- Builds endurance
- Stabilization of the spine
- Greater awareness of posture
- Improves physical coordination and balance
- Helps prevent musculoskeletal injuries.

CHAPTER

22

Rood's Approach

Divya Midha

HISTORY

Using the words of Miss Rood (1966) *"The following hypothesis is an attempt at a brief total concept of the reactions of the body which might affect the evaluations of patients and the clinical application of therapy".* Her approach deals with the activation or de-activation of developing somatic, autonomic and mental functions (Fig. 22.1).

An approach for the treatment of neurological dysfunction was proposed by Margeret S Rood in the year 1950. Margaret S Rood was formally educated in occupational and physical therapy. Her

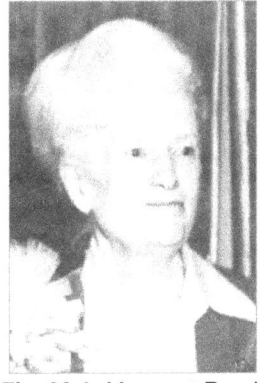

Fig. 22.1: Margaret Rood.

theory originated in the 1940s and underwent many revisions before she died. The work of Margaret Rood evolved from developmental and neurophysiological literature of 1930s. Because of this literature, it was believed that motor output is dependent upon sensory input, motor response follow a normal developmental sequence and psychic, somatic, and autonomic functions are also interrelated.

Rood's basic assumption rested upon the belief that motor functions are inseparable from sensory mechanisms. Therefore, sensory factors and their relationship to motor functions assumed a major role in the analysis of dysfunction and in the application of this treatment.

In the Roods approach, muscle groups are categorized according to the type of work they perform and their responses to the specific stimuli. Light work refers to the movement with reciprocal inhibition of antagonist muscles. This may occur in voluntary movement or autonomic nervous system action. The light work muscles (mobilizers) are primarily the flexors and adductors used for skilled movement patterns. Heavy work is defined as holding or co-contraction of muscles that are antagonists in normal movement and that are used to provide a stable support to the joint in a fixed position. The heavy work muscles (stabilizers) are principally the extensors and abductors used for postural support. Some muscles perform both light and heavy work functions.

Using these concepts of light and heavy work, Rood outlined the normal developmental sequence by using the following order of activation of muscles groups.

STAGE-I: RECIPROCAL INNERVATION OR MOBILITY

It is reciprocal and alternate movement of the limbs through full range while fully supported in the supine, roll over and prone positions. For developing voluntary movement control, the reflex activation of movement patterns is done via reciprocal innervations of the joints till the control is developed without reflex, e.g. stroking at palm of the hand or sole of the feet promotes crossed movement of extremities over anterior surface of body. Rood called it as supine withdrawal and she implemented it for the treatment of patients who had extremities dominated by the extension.

STAGE-II: COINNERVATION OR CO-CONTRACTION

Defined as simultaneous contractions of antagonists and agonists, working together to stabilize and maintaining posture of the body, e.g. maintaining posture of neck by co-contractions, prone on elbows, all on fours and standing. Neck and head contraction can be achieved by placing the patient in prone lying position on the bed or supporting surface with head and neck hanging down without support over the edge down towards the floor. Any visual or auditory stimuli can be given or any activity can be provided for promoting head righting. Co-contraction should be avoided in severe head injury cases.

STAGE-III: HEAVY WORK—MOVEMENT SUPERIMPOSED ON MOBILITY

It is defined as movement of proximal limb segments with the distal ends of limbs fixed on the base of support. It includes weight shifts on the floor, e.g. partial weight shifting in prone on elbows, all on fours, to and fro rocking that later on can be promoted to crawling in different directions. Weight shifts also make an individual to be prepared for the equilibrium responses. Mobility superimposed on stability is achieved by heavy work muscles or proximal muscles, i.e. deep tonic extensors of neck and trunk, scapular muscles, pelvis (abductors and external rotators), etc. Heavy work muscles are mainly composed of red fibers (aerobic), run obliquely, have rich blood supply with low metabolic cost. However, concept of mobility superimposed over stability is yet controversial as some studies state that proximal and distal controls develop separately, e.g. in case of upper extremity fine motor skills can be developed separately even without scapular stability.

STAGE-IV: SKILL

Skilled work with emphasis on the movement of distal portions of the body that requires control from the highest cortical level. It is produced by the light work muscles. Light work muscles are responsible for carrying out phasic movements, i.e. repetitive or rhythmic patterns of distal musculature. They are composed of white fibers (anaerobic) and have high metabolic cost. They are primarily adductors, flexors and internal rotators.

Along with the concept of light and heavy work in the developmental sequence, the Rood approach identified two major sequences in motor development that are distinctly different, but inseparable due to their interaction. The two sequences are those of skeletal functions and vital functions. The skeletal functions include activities of the head, neck, trunk, and extremities while the vital functions include vegetative, respiratory, and speech activities.

Rood also believed that a voluntary motor act is based on inherent reflexes and on modification of those reflexes at higher centers. Therefore, she begun therapy by eliciting motor responses on a reflex level and incorporating developmental patterns to enhance the motor response.

Stimulation of the sensory receptors is done in the sequence of normal development from the most primitive reflexes to the skill level. The purpose of treatment is to restore that component in the sequence in the manner in which would be normally acquired. Therefore, the Rood approach to treatment is proposed to be applicable to any type of neurologic dysfunction at any age.

SEQUENCE OF GROSS MOTOR DEVELOPMENT

1. Supine Withdrawal

Description: Flexed posture, heavy work of trunk, neck and all the proximal joints, reciprocal innervation, movement occurs towards t10 vertebra (Fig. 22.2).

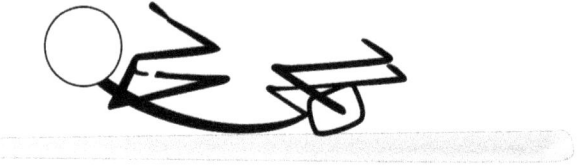

Fig. 22.2: Supine withdrawal.

2. Roll Over

Description: Flexion of upper and lower extremities, phasic movement pattern (Fig. 22.3).

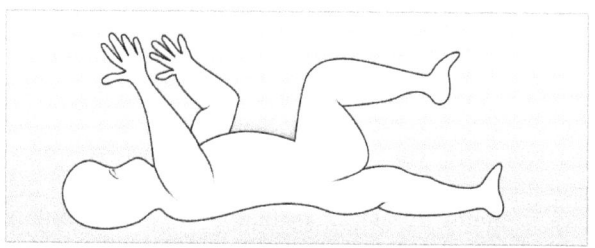

Fig. 22.3: Roll over.

3. Pivot Pattern

Description: Total extension and bilateral holding of proximal extensors, reciprocal innervation pattern (Fig. 22.4).

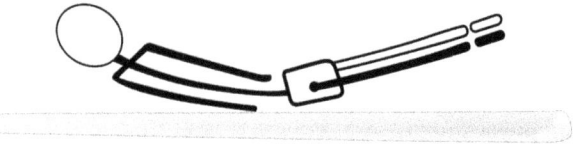

Fig. 22.4: Pivot pattern.

4. Co-contraction Neck

Description: Co-contraction of neck extensors, thoracic extension (Fig. 22.5).

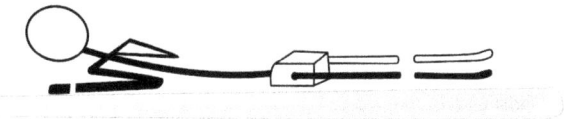

Fig. 22.5: Co-contraction neck.

5. Forearm Support

Description: Scapular co-contraction, glenohumeral joint co-contraction (Fig. 22.6).

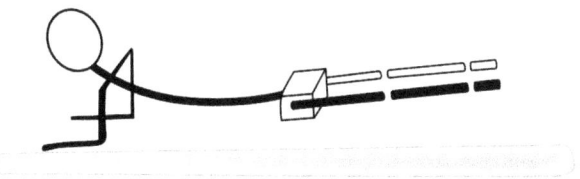

Fig. 22.6: Forearm support.

6. All on Fours

Description: Weight bearing on both upper limbs and lower limbs. Weight shifts forward-backward, sideways (Fig. 22.7).

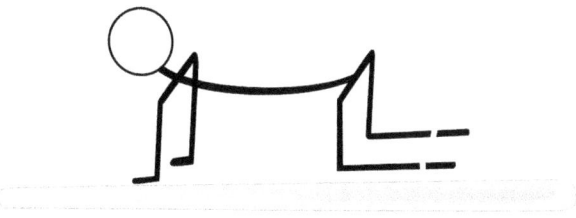

Fig. 22.7: All on four.

7. Standing

Description: Static weight bearing on bilateral limbs (Fig. 22.8).

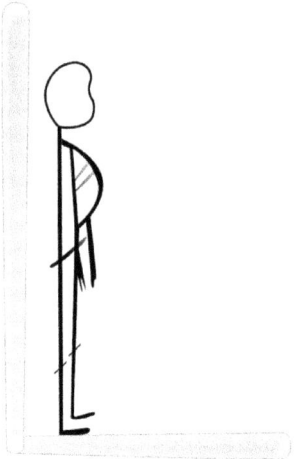

Fig. 22.8: Standing.

8. Walking

Description: Dynamic weight bearing on both the lower limbs (Fig. 22.9).

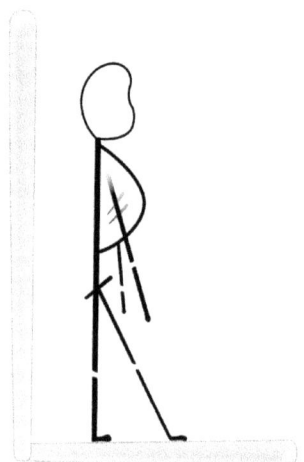

Fig. 22.9: Walking.

MUSCLE TONE

Muscle tone involves active tension and passive (resting) intrinsic viscoelastic tone. Human resting tone was defined as passive tone/tension of the skeletal muscle that derives from intrinsic viscoelastic properties, i.e. resting muscle tone is viscoelastic stiffness without contractile activity.

Any neurological insult is associated with wide range of tone abnormalities with which execution of any movement becomes difficult. Two commonest tone abnormalities associated with neurological disorders is hypertonicity and hypotonicity.

Hypertonia is a condition in which there is increased muscle tone. Arms, legs or any affected part becomes stiff and offers too much resistance against movement on passive elongation. Abnormal high tone causes malalignment of the trunk and limbs. Excessive shortening of muscles may cause a joint to become frozen and subsequent deformity thus interfering with the ADL's, e.g. if hypertonia affects lower limbs, walking becomes difficult as it becomes difficult for the body to react quickly to regain balance.

Hypertonicity or high tone is increased resistance to the passive elongation of the muscle. It causes greater impairment, worst function; low health related quality of life. In addition to increased rest activity, abnormal patterns of muscle activation such as spastic co-contractions may contribute to disability.

Hypotonia is described as reduced resistance to passive range of motion in joints. A hypotonic muscle lacks ability to sustain postural control and movement against gravity. Such patients exhibit poor control of movements and delayed motor skills.

Primary goal of treatment for patients with neurological dysfunction having tone abnormalities is "normalization of tone". Goal can be achieved completely through various sensory inputs for eliciting muscle contraction or inhibiting muscle tone.

ROODS TREATMENT TECHNIQUES

Every patient has different characteristics so it is a great challenge for the physical therapist to select methods most efficient for each patient's needs. Appropriate selection of the treatment methods and techniques depends upon the understanding of many aspects, such as:

- The neurophysiological bases of each method
- The biomechanical influencing of the applied technique on the treated body part(s), segment(s), or body as a whole.

To initiate a movement response technique should be focused on increasing the neuronal activity, i.e. facilitation and to decrease a movement response we should focus on decreasing the neuronal activity, i.e. inhibition. The sensory stimulation techniques can be used separately or can also be grouped as per the receptors required to be activated. The nature of stimulation (intensity of the stimulus, duration and frequency of the treatment technique can be adjusted according to the individual needs of the patient.

Facilitation Techniques

Facilitation techniques are used by providing sensory stimulation to specific muscle groups. They are categorized as tactile stimuli, thermal stimuli and propioceptive stimuli.

Light Touch

Light touch or stroking of the skin done is at the dorsum of hand, sole of feet and palmar surface of the hand. It promotes withdrawal of the limb, causing shortening of whole extremity producing flexion of all the joints of the extremity. Stroking activates A-sensory fibers which further activate withdrawal reflex by activating phasic response of the muscles. Frequency of strokes is 2 per second and can be applied for 3–5 times.

Brushing

The brushing technique is one of the specific method of stimulation to help the brain to organize sensory information. The brushing technique is delivered through a soft camel hair paint brush that can be attached to a hand held battery operated mixer to produce a high frequency and high intensity stimulus. Brush should not be kept vertical rather it should be held tilted to avoid hair pulling. Brushing causes stimulation of C-sensory fibers. According to Rood, technique reaches its maximum facilitative state after 30–40 minutes of stimulation, though some studies state that brushing do cause immediate effect with the therapeutic effect lasting just for 35–40 seconds.

Fast brushing over areas such as pinna of the ear should be avoided as it causes activation of parasympathetic fibers thus it may interfere with the cardiorespiratory functions such as slowing down of heart rate, constriction of bronchial muscles with activation of smooth muscles. It should also be avoided over lower lumbar area at the level of S2-S4 as it may induce bladder dysfunction causing urination.

Thermal Stimulation

Thermal stimulation by means of icing was developed by Rood for eliciting motor patterns. Rood used repetitive stimulus with the help of an ice cube. Ice cube is rubbed with pressure for 3–5 seconds in the form of quick swipes. Once the stimulus is given initially it may develop a phasic withdrawal reflex. It causes stimulation of exteroreceptors and propioceptors and also a brief cortical arousal due to activation of reticular activating system. Two different types of icing are A-icing and C-icing based on the type of fibers needed to be stimulated.

A-icing: A-icing is done by means three quick strokes done with an ice cube over palm of the hands. Sole of foot or dorsal surface of the hand to evoke flexor response of the limb generating withdrawal reflex. Many researches have been done on the facilitatory responses generated by means of A-icing. Stimulation of the diaphragm and muscles of inspiration by application of the icing along the rib cage at T7-T9 level, touching the lips stimulates mouth opening, application of ice to the tongue facilitates mouth closure. Swallowing can also be initiated by application of quick ice strokes over sternal notch.

C-icing: C-icing is also done with the help of an ice cube but stimulus is relatively of high threshold than the A-icing. It is accomplished by placing and keeping the ice cube on the targeted area for 3–6 seconds. It causes activation of the C-sensory fibers. Icing is contraindicated in the distribution of posterior primary rami along the lower lumbar area as it may cause sympathetic nervous system fight and flight response. Icing is also contraindicated in patients with circulatory disturbances, e.g. Reynauld's phenomena. Icing should be avoided in the hypersensitive areas like pinna of the ear as it may induce vagal responses along with the cardiorespiratory disturbances. It should also be avoided over areas like forehead, upper portion of lips and midline of trunk as there is higher concentration of pain fibers over these areas.

Quick Stretch

Quick stretch is administered for initiating muscle contraction. It is administered by providing submaximal stretch to the targeted muscle by keeping it in a maximally lengthened position. Excessive stretch should not be given as it may cause pain and cause withdrawal of the extremity. It can also be applied by the therapist by keeping fingertips to vigorously tap the skin over muscle or tendon while patient attempts to do the movement. Quick stretch is given via low threshold stimulus that activates immediate phasic response by activating stretch reflex facilitating agonists and inhibiting antagonists, producing a very short contraction or movement via Ia fibers of muscle spindle.

Vibration

High frequency vibration can be applied by a mechanical or an electrical vibrator over the muscle belly or over muscle tendon over a slightly stretched muscle. Though some researchers say that application of vibration stimulus over muscle tendon may cause unnecessary activation of the undesired muscles of surrounding areas. Excursion of such device is up to the depth of 1-2 mm. Vibration causes stimulation of Ia fibers of the muscle spindle, also providing repetitive mechanical stretch to the muscle fibers known as tonic vibratory reflex. Effect of vibration lasts for 30-60 seconds as long as stimulus is applied. Duration of the stimulus should be kept for 1-2 minutes longer than this duration can cause heat and friction causing potential tearing of the underlying skin.

Lot of researches has been done to find out the appropriate frequency of vibration stimulus for getting desirable response yet the matter is debatable. Trombly suggests 100 Hz to 300 Hz, Umphered and Mc Cormack say frequency over 200 Hz may cause damage to skin tissue and discomfort and pain to the muscle fibers.

Muscle Tapping

Muscle tapping facilitates muscle by initiating muscle contraction. It is done with the fingertips striking quickly at the muscle belly. Muscle tapping promotes contraction for very shorter duration by stimulating primary Ia fibers of the muscle spindle. Many researches have been conducted on the speed of muscle tapping and findings suggest that muscle tapping can cause radiation of the force to the unwanted muscles via bone if tap is given at higher intensity than the lower intensity.

Rood's Approach

Joint Distraction

This is administered by moving articular surfaces of the joint apart from each other. Joint distraction causes stimulation of the joint receptors located within the joint cavity as well as the surrounding structures of the joint. Joint distraction is applied by manually pulling both the articulating surfaces apart along the longitudinal axis of the bone.

Resistance

Resistance is provided to the ongoing movement or to promote co-contraction of the muscles. Co-contraction promotes postural stability as there occurs firing of the Golgi tendon organs (GTO) with significant increase in their firing as the amount of the resistance increases. Amount of motor unit firing is higher when muscle is loaded against resistance than without resistance this is known as overflow phenomena. Resistance also enhances kinesthetic awareness which further promotes motor learning.

Inhibition Techniques

Inhibition techniques are applied with the provision of the sensory stimuli for the longer duration. Inhibition techniques are used for the treatment of hypertonicity.

Slow Stroking

Slow and rhythmic stroking over distribution of posterior rami induces general relaxation. Slow stroking is applied on the whole back starting from occiput till coccyx along the vertebral musculature by using palm or fingers extended. Stimulus should be applied from occiput to coccyx and vice versa continuously for 3–5 minutes longer than this may cause rebound of autonomic responses. Therapist should not leave the contact with the skin by keeping one hand in contact with the skin as long as the stimulation is in process. Once the one hand is over the lowest lumbar area, the other hand should be placed over cervical region. Before concluding the stimulation therapist should not lift the hands. Any lubricant can also be used over the area to be treated and index and middle fingers are used over paravertebrally. Stroking should be avoided in the patients who have hypersensitivity over hair follicles.

Neutral Warmth

Neutral warmth is given by wrapping the body part to be inhibited for the duration of 3-5 minutes. Whole body relaxation can be induced by application of stimuli over distribution of posterior rami on the back. Neutral warmth can be given by a cotton flannel or fleece blanket or a down comforter for 10-15 minutes. Neutral warmth is applied with the temperature keeping more than the body temperature to avoid rebound effect in 2-3 hours. Effect of neutral warmth can be enhanced with the application of prolong pressure that can be applied manually, perpendicular to the longitudinal axis to the muscle tendon or mechanically with the help of various objects like cone in the hand for inhibiting finger flexion, platform shoes for inhibiting plantar flexion. Elastic bandages and air splints can also be used for inhibiting hypertonicity. Prolong pressure causes activation of the Golgi tendon organs (GTO), that causes inhibition of the agonist muscle, pacinian corpuscles.

Prolong Icing

With prolong icing neural transmission of impulses is reduced in both afferents and efferents. Prolong icing can be given in the form of ice massage. It reduces hypertonicity and induces relaxation in the agonist muscles. Prolong icing can be applied for 10-15 minutes for inducing inhibiting effect. Prolong icing can also be applied with an ice pack to be placed over the area to be inhibited. Prolong icing causes inhibition of the stretch reflex by inhibiting tone of agonist muscles.

Vestibular Stimuli

Vestibular system is responsible for maintenance of balance as it relays information about the orientation of head and neck and linear acceleration in the space. Vestibular system has connections with auditory, visual, propioceptive and motor system. Slow, rhythmic rolling can be done by the therapist by moving the patient from supine lying to side lying by taking the patient comfortable supine lying with proper pillow support under head and neck and below knees. Therapist supports the patient at the shoulder and hip. Constant, slow and rhythmic rocking movement cause general inhibition of the total body response. Stimulation should be stopped if undesired responses are generated.

Prolong Stretch

Prolong stretch is given manually for inhibiting hypertonicity. Extremity should be kept in maximally lengthened positioned for 20-30 seconds. Prolong stretch can be given manually by the external force applied by the therapist or by means of mechanical devices as splints by keeping the muscles in stretched position for several hours to several weeks. Mechanical stretch causes structural changes in the skeletal muscle promoting growth of sarcomeres, changing viscoelastic properties of muscle disrupting actin-myosin cross bridges thus making the muscle to be less sensitive to the stretch force. It also reduces stiffness landed due to hypertonicity in the nearby connective tissues.

Joint Approximation

Joint approximation is done by gently moving articular surfaces of the joint close to each other. It causes inhibition of the spasticity and also improves propioception in the joint cavity and the surrounding surfaces.

Tendon Pressure

Many cutaneous receptors are rapidly adapting hence maintained stimulus may cause inhibition of the motor responses. Maintained pressure can be used for therapeutic purpose to alter the motor responses. Tendon pressure can be applied manually or mechanically with the help of cone pads, orthokinetic cuff, developed by Blashy and Fuchs. Deep and maintained pressure causes activation of the pacinian corpuscles. Tendon pressure is applied over musculotendinous junctions over insertion of the muscles. Flexors of hand and wrist can be inhibiting by application of prolong pressure over tendinous insertion of muscles and keeping the muscles in maximally lengthened position.

CHAPTER 23

Bobath Concept/ Neurodevelopmental Treatment

Krishna N Sharma

The Bobath concept is a problem solving approach to the assessment and treatment of individuals with disturbances of function, movement and postural control due to a lesion of the central nervous system.
—**IBITA**

HISTORY

- *Dr Karel Bobath*, a medical doctor was born in Berlin, Germany in 1906 (Fig. 23.1).
- *Mrs Berta Ottilie Busse*, a remedial gymnast was born in Berlin, Germany in 1907 (Fig. 23.1).
- Both shifted to London in 1938 and got married in 1941.
- Mrs Bobath was asked to treat a famous portrait painter and a stroke patient in 1943, and observed that handling has an important role in managing spasticity, stiffness and movement control.
- Her observations gave her a spark and her constant observation of the patients during 1945–1975 gave the origin to the *Bobath concept*.
- After developing the techniques, the Bobath couple presented a scientific rationale based on the theories of that time.
- The first article describing the Bobath approach was published in 1948.

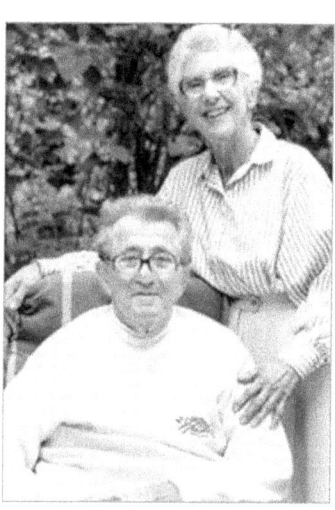

Fig. 23.1: Dr. Karel Bobath and Mrs Berta Bobath.

- *Mrs Bobath* graduated as a physiotherapist from the Chartered Society of Physiotherapy in 1950.
- The Bobath couple founded *Western Cerebral Palsy Centre* in 1951.
- They founded *The Bobath Centre* in 1975.
- *International Bobath Instructors Training Association (IBITA)* was formed in 1984.
- *British Bobath Tutors Association (BBTA)* was formed in 1994.
- Bobath concept is also known as *Neurodevelopmental Treatment (NDT)*.

CONCEPTS
Old Concept
The old concept was based on *reflex hierarchical theory*—the most accepted motor control theory of that time. It says that movements elicit through the reflexes in the spinal cord and any lesion to the pyramidal tract causes loss of inhibitory control on the reflexes and thus causes spasticity.

Current Concept
The current concept (and it is still developing) is more focused towards the neuroplasticity. Now the Bobath therapists believe that:
- The CNS is a complex organization consisting of "systems and subsystem".
- Movement control is dependent upon and intact, integrated neurological and musculoskeletal system.
- Selective movement control of the trunk and the limbs interact with and are interdependent with a postural control mechanism.
- The CNS can adapt and change its structural organization and thus the manipulation of afferent input can influence its structural organization.
- The treatment should be focused on learning motor control instead of compensatory actions.

IMPORTANT CONCEPTS
Requirements for Normal Movement
- Normal muscle tone

- Normal postural responses
- Normal motor patterns and coordination.

Components of Motor Disturbance in Adult Hemiplegia
- Abnormal Tone
    - *Flaccidity:* Hypotonicity during the acute phase
    - *Spasticity:* Hypertonicity after the acute phase
        i. *Placing response:* If a spastic limb is moved passively, the muscle tone follows the movement. That is why during passive movement if the therapist suddenly removes the hand, the patient's limb remains in the same position for some time.
        ii. *Associated reactions:* Strong efforts elicit hypertonicity and nonfunctional involuntary change in the position of the limbs (abnormal flexion pattern in upper limb and extension pattern in lower limb).
- Loss of postural control
- Abnormal coordination:
    - Disturbed agonist-synergist-antagonist coordination
    - Disturbed sequence of muscles contraction
    - Disturbed timing of muscles contraction.
- Abnormal functional performance.

PRINCIPLES
- Treatment should be individualized
- Efforts should be made to normalize tone
- Any activity or movement that increases the muscle tone and elicit any abnormal motor response (postural, primitive reflex patterns and mass synergies) during the treatment should be avoided
- Emphasis should be on developing normal patterns of posture and movement
- Efforts should be made to normalize the sensory and perceptual experiences through tactile and kinesthetic stimulation
- Treatment is aimed at promoting quality of movement and functional performance.

ASSESSMENT

The therapist uses observations, handling, and interview to identify and assess:
- Presence and distribution of abnormal tone and motor pattern
- Deficits in normal motor responses
- Ability of performing functional movement patterns.

TECHNIQUES

- Handling (key points of control)
  - Inhibition techniques
  - Facilitation techniques
- Guided movement
- Rhythmic rotation
- Proprioceptive inputs
- Exteroceptive inputs
- Verbal commands.

CHAPTER 24

Brunnstrom Movement Therapy

Krishna N Sharma

Signe Brunnstrom—a Swedish female physical therapist (Fig. 24.1), said that during the normal stages of development, spinal cord and brainstem reflexes modifies and are rearranged into voluntary movement by the influence of higher motor centers; and since the reflexes in hemiplegic patients represent normal stages of development, these can be used to regain the motor abilities. So in her approach she encouraged development of flexor and extensor synergies during early recovery.

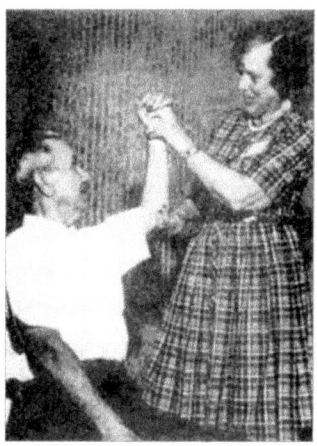

Fig. 24.1: Signe Brunnstrom (right).

BASIC CONCEPTS
(Adopted From Brunnstrom, 1956 and 1970)

1. In normal motor development, spinal cord and brainstem reflexes become modified and their components rearranged into purposeful movement through the influence of higher centers. Because reflexes and whole-limb movement patterns are normal stages of development and because stroke appears to result in "development in reverse" reflexes and primitive movement patterns should be used to facilitate the recovery of voluntary movement poststroke. It may well be that a subcortical motion synergy which can be elicited on a reflex basis may serve as a wedge by means of which a limited amount of willed movement may be learned.
2. Proprioceptive and exteroceptive stimuli can be used to evoke desired motion or tonal changes.

3. Recovery of voluntary movement poststroke proceeds in sequence from mass, flexor or extensor limb synergy movement patterns to movements that combine features of the two patterns, and finally to voluntary discrete movements of each joint.
4. Newly produced, correct motions must be practiced to be learned.
5. Practice within the context of daily activities enhances the learning process.

EVALUATION

In Brunnstrom approach, the therapist does the following 6 evaluations in the patient.
1. *Sensory evaluation:* The patient's sensory status.
2. *Tonic reflexes:* The effect of tonic reflexes on the patient's movement.
3. *Associated reactions:* The effect of associated reactions on the patient's movement.
4. *Stages of motor recovery:* The level of recovery of voluntary motor control.
5. *Speed test:* To assess the spasticity during the recovery stages in the patients with active ROM.
6. *Limb synergies:* Assessment of basic limb synergies.

Sensory Evaluation

- *Touch sensation:* The patient sits on a chair is blindfolded. The therapist touches palmar aspect of the finger tips with a rubber end of a pencil and asks to tell which fingertip is touched.
- *Sole sensation:* The patient sits or lies down blindfolded. The therapist touches and/or presses sole of the foot and asks to the patient if his sole is being touched or pressed. If the patient says yes, then the therapist asks the location on the sole.
- *Joint position sense:* The patient sits on a chair is blindfolded. The therapist supports the affected upper limb and moves to different positions asking the patient to move another upper limb to the same position.

Tonic Reflexes

- *Asymmetric tonic neck reflex (ATNR):* Head rotation to one side cause extension of upper and lower limb of the side of rotation and flexion of the upper and lower limb of another side.

- *Symmetric tonic neck reflex (STNR):* Passive flexion of the neck causes flexion of the upper limbs and extension of the lower limbs. Extension of the neck causes extension of the upper limbs and flexion of the lower limbs.
- *Tonic labyrinthine reflex (TLR):* Supine position facilitates extension, and the prone lying position facilitates flexion.
- *Tonic lumbar reflex:* Rotation of the upper trunk (with respect to the pelvis) to one side causes flexion of upper limb and extension of lower limb of the side of rotation; and extension of upper limb and flexion of lower limb of the another side.
- *Tonic thumb reflex:* When the affected upper limb is elevated above horizontal with forearm supination, thumb extension is facilitated.

Associated Reactions
- *Souques' phenomenon:* Elevation of the affected arm in pronation above the horizontal causes an extension and abduction response of the fingers.
- *Raimiste's phenomenon:* Resistance applied to abduction or adduction of the normal lower extremity produces a similar reaction in the affected limb.
- *Homolateral limb Synkineses:* Flexion of the affected upper limb elicits flexion of the affected lower limb.

Stages of Motor Recovery
- **Stage 1:** Flaccidity with no voluntary movement.
- **Stage 2:** Spasticity is present but is not marked. Development of basic limb synergy. No voluntary movement.
- **Stage 3:** Maximum spasticity. Development of limb synergy voluntarily.
- **Stage 4:** Spasticity begins to decrease. Voluntary movements deviating from synergies. Patient is now able to do the following:
  - Placing the hand behind the body.
  - Alternative pronation-supination with the elbow at 90° flexion.
  - Elevation of the arm to a forward horizontal position.
- **Stage 5:** Spasticity is waning. Voluntary independence from basic synergies. Patient is now able to do the following:
  - Bringing hand over the head.
  - Arm raising to a side horizontal position.
  - Alternative pronation-supination with the elbow extended.

- **Stage 6:** Voluntary isolated joint movement with almost normal coordination.

Speed Test

The patient sits on a chair without armrest with the back and head as erect as possible. The therapist instructs patient to move the hand from lap to chin (requiring complete range of elbow flexion) and chin to lap repeatedly for 5 seconds; and move the hand from lap to opposite knee (requiring full range of elbow extension) and opposite knee to lap repeatedly for 5 seconds. This test is done by both the affected and unaffected arm.

Limb Synergies

Flexor Synergy of Upper Limb
- Scapula: Retraction and depression
- Shoulder: Flexion, abduction (weakest component), and external rotation (weakest component)
- Elbow: Flexion to acute angle (strongest component)
- Forearm: Supination
- Wrist and fingers: Variable. Most commonly flexed.

Extensor Synergy of Upper Limb
- Scapula: Protraction
- Shoulder: Extension, adduction (strongest component), and internal rotation
- Elbow: Extension (weakest component)
- Forearm: Pronation (strongest component)
- Wrist and fingers: Variable. Most commonly flexed.

Flexor Synergy of Lower Limb
- Hip: Flexion (strongest component), abduction (weakest component), external rotation (weakest component)
- Knee: Flexion to about 90°
- Ankle: Dorsiflexion and inversion
- Toes: Dorsiflexion.

Extensor Synergy of Lower Limb
- Hip: Extension, adduction (strongest component), internal rotation (weakest component)
- Knee: Extension (strongest component)

- Ankle: Plantar flexion, inversion
- Toes: Plantar flexion.

TREATMENT PRINCIPLES

- Use developmental recovery sequence. Progress the treatment developmentally, i.e. from reflex to voluntary, and from voluntary to function.
- In the absence of motion, facilitate movement through sensory stimulation e.g. reflexes, associated reactions, proprioceptive and/or exteroceptive facilitation.
    - The elicited reflex responses and associated reactions should be combined with the patient's voluntary effort to move. It produces semi-voluntary movement, which allows the patient to experience the sensory feedback associated with movement.
    - Proprioceptive (resistance) and exteroceptive stimuli (tactile stimulation) assist in eliciting movement. The exteroceptive stimuli facilitate only the muscles related to the stimulated area, whereas proprioceptive stimuli facilitate other muscles too by producing an associated reaction/patterned response.
- When voluntary effort produces, ask the patient to hold the position (isometric contraction) and move voluntarily (initially eccentric, then concentric contraction).
- When even only partial movement is possible, reversal of movement from flexion to extension is stressed within each treatment session.
- Facilitation is reduced or dropped out as soon as the patient shows evidence of volitional control. First of all, reflexes that are the most primitive are dropped out of treatment and tactile stimulation (exteroceptive stimulation) are eliminated at the last. No primitive reflexes, including associated reactions are used beyond stage 3.
- Willed movement (a movement that the patient is trying to accomplish, e.g. reaching for a glass) should be emphasized to break the linkages between parts of the synergies.
- Once the correct movement is elicited, the patient should repeat it many times and functional activities should be included in this practice.

CHAPTER 25

Vojta Therapy

Krishna N Sharma

The basic movement patterns are programmed genetically in each individual's central nervous system.
— **Professor Vojta**

HISTORY

- It was developed between 1950 and 1970 by Dr Vaclàv Vojta, a neurologist born on the 12th July 1917 in Mokrosuky, Bohemia, Czech Republic (Fig. 25.1).
- Dr Vojta observed that the cerebral palsy children respond to certain stimuli in certain body positions with recurring motor reactions in the trunk and the extremities.
- Dr Vojta immigrated to Germany in August 1968 and worked at the University Orthopaedic Clinic, Cologne, as well as at the Munich Children's Centre.
- He started teaching Vojta therapy in 1990.

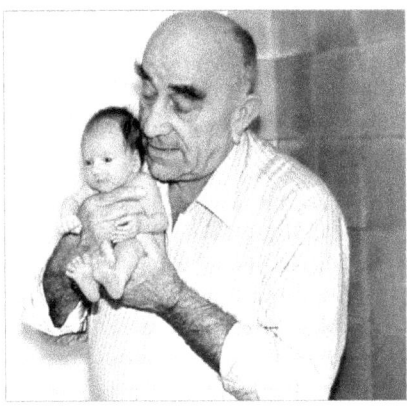

Fig. 25.1: Dr Vaclàv Vojta.

PRINCIPLES AND FUNDAMENTALS OF VOJTA THERAPY

1. The reflex locomotion is achieved by applying pressure on trigger zones with body in certain position
2. Vojta therapy does not teach or train normal movement processes
3. Vojta therapy activates natural and innate capabilities by sending stimuli to the brain
4. Vojta therapy improves postural regulation, uprighting the body against gravity, and phasic mobility (goal-directed movement)
5. Reflex locomotion can be activated in the patients of any age group
6. The effects of Vojta therapy depends on the type and extend of illness
7. Patient attendants play an integral role in administering the exercises.

PRINCIPLE OF REFLEX LOCOMOTION

The Vojta therapy is based on the principle of *reflex locomotion*. According to Prof Vojta, there are few reflex points (*trigger zones*) in the body that activate certain muscle groups when stimulated by applying pressure. It also regulates breathing and increases mental activity.

The therapist starts with thorough assessment of static states, i.e. head lifting in prone, rolling, side sitting, erect sitting, creeping, standing and walking. Then the therapist places the patient in one of the three basic positions (prone, side lying, supine) with specific initial angular position of the body segments, applies pressure and pull in the joint, activates trigger zones and provides resistance against the motion. It initiates certain movement complexes (coordination complexes)—*reflex creeping* and *reflex rolling*.

Reflex Creeping

Reflex creeping is initiated in prone position and it produces a kind of creeping movement. The patient is placed in prone position with head slightly rotated. The upper/lower extremities on the side of head rotation (towards face) are called *facial upper extremity* and *facial lower extremity*. The extremities of another side (towards occiput) are called *occipital upper extremity* and *occipital lower extremity*. The therapist chooses *initial position* and *trigger zones* according to

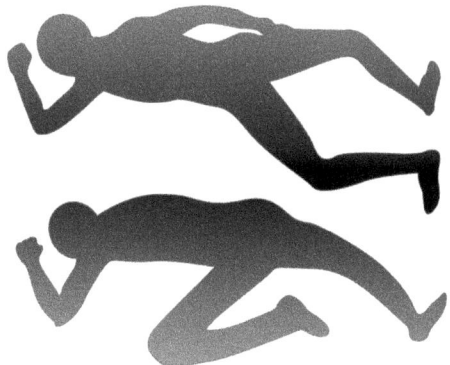

Fig. 25.2: Reflex creeping sequence (*Source:* Vojta's website).

required *anticipatory movements*. On stimulation, the movement occurs in *crossed pattern* where one side of upper extremity moves simultaneously with another side of lower extremity (Fig. 25.2).

Effects of Reflex Creeping
- Activation of the muscular support and uprighting mechanisms
- Activation of the respiratory, abdominal, and pelvic floor muscles
- Activation of the sphincters of the bladder and bowel
- Activation of swallowing
- Activation of eye movements.

Reflex Rolling

Reflex rolling is initiated in from supine lying position and it progresses into quadrupedal gait (creeping in quadrupedal position) via a side lying position. Reflex rolling has two phases—*Phase 1* and *Phase 2*.

In *Phase 1*, the therapist positions the patient in supine lying with neck rotated and resists neck rotation with stimulation of *breast zone* to achieve rotation to side.

In *Phase 2*, the therapist positions the patient in side-lying and stimulates various *trigger zones* of upper and lower extremities to achieve quadrupedal gait (Fig. 25.3).

INDICATIONS

Thought it can be applied in adults too, the Vojta therapy is preferred to be used in children with movement disorders due to

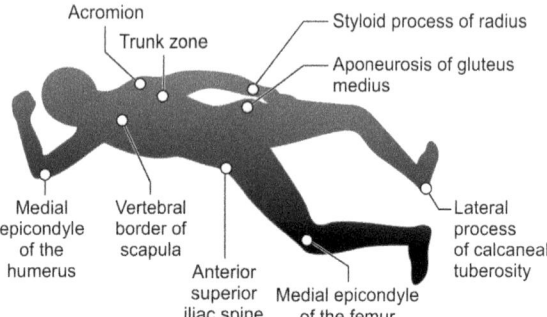

Fig. 25.3: Trigger zones (*Source:* Vojta's website).

nervous system disorders, myopathies, orthopedic conditions and other illnesses, e.g. dysplasia, dislocations, deformities, breathing problems, dysphagia, etc.

CONTRAINDICATIONS

- Fever
- Inflammatory conditions
- Recent vaccination
- With caution in the cases of pregnancy, osteoporosis, osteogenesis imperfecta, heart disease, etc.

CHAPTER 26

Motor Relearning Program

Krishna N Sharma

"Motor Relearning Program" or MRP was developed by the duo of Australian physiotherapists "Janet Carr (Fig. 26.1) and Roberta Shepherd" (1987) for the stroke patients. This program emphasizes motor relearning by practicing task-specific motor activities.

THEORETICAL BASIS

This program is based on the systemic model of motor control and system theory of motor development. It suggests that the order of sections is not important and mastery of a section is not necessary before going onto another section.

Carr and Shepherd believed that the motor behaviors emerge as a result of context or regulatory conditions in the environment. The stroke patients lose the ability to generate appropriate models of action. It leads to stereotypic movement patters as the result of compensatory strategies the patient use to perform a task or a movement.

On this theoretical basis, *Carr and Shepherd* discouraged the early use of compensatory strategies and suggested to teach the

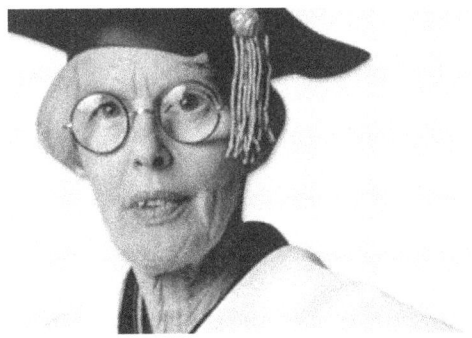

Fig. 26.1: Janet Carr.

patients how to avoid abnormal compensation for weak muscles. They emphasized motor relearning by practicing task-specific motor activities and focused on the interaction between the performer and the environment. That is why in MRP, the patients practice movement patterns in context of tasks, rather than exercises.

ASSESSMENT

In this program, the therapist analyzes each task separately and identifies the components the patient is unable to perform well. Then the therapist trains the patient in those identified components of the task, and ensures carryover of this training during daily activities.

The motor relearning program (MRP) is a task specific training where the therapist assesses and trains the patient in seven different task of daily life. *Carr and Shepherd* classified the functional daily activities in 7 categories:

1. Upper limb function
2. Oro-facial function
3. Sitting up from supine
4. Sitting
5. Standing up and sitting down
6. Standing
7. Walking

STEPS FOR INTERVENTION

1. Analysis of task
   a. Observation
   b. Comparison
   c. Analysis
2. Practice of missing components
   a. Identification of goals
   b. Instruction
   c. Practice with verbal and visual feedback and manual guidance
3. Practice of task
   a. Identification of goals
   b. Instruction
   c. Practice with verbal and visual feedback and manual guidance

d. Progression
   e. Reevaluation
4. Transference of learning
   a. Opportunity to practice in context
   b. Consistency of practice and positive reinforcement
   c. Organization of self-monitored practice
   d. Structured and stimulating learning environment
   e. Involvement of relatives and staff.

EQUIPMENT
- Objects that can be used as normally operative regulatory conditions for tasks.
- Unnecessary equipment
   - Parallel bars and canes
   - Ankle splints/braces.

PRECAUTIONS
- The program should be designed for the individual patient and new tasks should be continually added according to the patient's emerging capacities.
- The therapist himself/herself should perform the task for visual demonstration and should focus on one or two most important components.
- Excessive physical handling should be avoided as a technique to teach patients the model of action.
- Verbal instruction should be minimal.
- The practice should be consistent.
- The therapist should give accurate, timely feedback about the quality of performance to the patient. It helps the patient to learn which strategies to repeat and which ones to avoid.

LIMITATIONS
- The patients with severe cognitive deficits cannot be treated as it focuses on active learning.
- Since spasticity is not considered as a significant residual problem of stroke, no management is recommended to reduce abnormal muscle tone.

CHAPTER 27

Proprioceptive Neuromuscular Facilitation

Kuki Bordoloi, Manisha Uttam, Harshita Yadav

DEFINITIONS

Kabat (1951): "PNF is a technique of treatment by neuromuscular facilitation using proprioceptive sensation with philosophy that all human being have untapped existing potential."

"Proprioceptive neuromuscular facilitation (PNF): It is an approach to therapeutic exercise that combines functionally based diagonal patterns of movement with techniques of neuromuscular facilitation to evoke motor responses and improve neuromuscular control and function."

"PNF is a motor learning approach used in neuromotor development training to improve motor function and facilitate maximum muscular contraction."

HISTORY

The term *Proprioceptive Facilitation* developed by *Dr Herman Kabat*—a neurophysiologist and physician in the early 1940's (Fig. 27.1). *Dorthy Voss* (1954)—a physiotherapist added the word *'Neuromuscular.' Dr Kabat* was influenced by 'Sister Elizabeth Kenny'—a nurse who used to use specific stretching and strengthening activities on polio patients. *Dr Kabat* started working on this with integration of *Sir Charles Sherrington's* work and lastly developed this treatment approach.

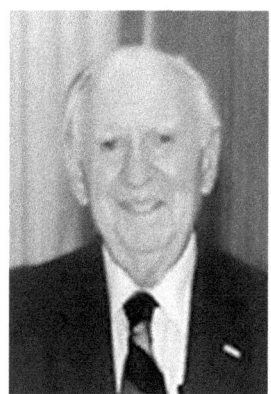

Fig. 27.1: Dr Herman Kabat.

PHILOSOPHY

It is a positive approach in which the patient hidden potential is stimulated by using intensive training. The treatment strategy includes the functional approach in which patient are given tasks which are successfully achieved by them without any pain to regain their highest functional level. The patient treatment includes emotional, physical and environmental aspects.

Proprioceptive neuromuscular facilitation (PNF) is started with a *positive approach*. The achievable tasks which are set up for success without pain are given for treatment. *Functional approach* is used to get highest functional level.

Potential is mobilized by using intensive training. The patient is treated as a whole including his/her emotional, personal, physical and environmental aspects. Motor control and learning principles are used.

AIMS

- To increase joint range of motion (ROM)
- To improve functional stability
- To improve motor control during movements
- To enhance motor co-ordination
- To induce relaxation
- To decrease muscle fatigue
- To decrease pain
- To increase muscle strength and endurance
- To initiate and teach a motion
- To promote functional movements.

PRINCIPLES OF PNF

There are 11 principles of PNF:

Principle 1: All human beings have potentials that are not fully developed.

Principle 2: Normal motor development proceeds in a cervico-caudal and proximal-distal direction.

Principle 3: Early motor behavior is dominated by reflex activity. Mature motor behavior is reinforced or supported by postural reflex mechanisms.

Principle 4: The growth of motor behavior has cyclic trends as evidenced by shifts between flexor and extensor dominance.

Principle 5: Goal-directed activity is made up of reversing movements.

Principle 6: Normal movement and posture depend on "synergism" and a balanced interaction of antagonists.

Principle 7: Developing motor behavior is expressed in an orderly sequence of total patterns of movement and posture.

Principle 8: Normal motor development has an orderly sequence but lacks a step-by-step quality; overlapping occurs.

Principle 9: Improvement of motor ability depends on motor learning.

Principle 10: Frequency of stimulation and repetition of activity are used for the promotion and retention of motor learning.

Principle 11: Goal-directed activities are used to hasten learning.

BASIC PROCEDURES

There are 10 components of the basic procedure of PNF, which are used together in several ways depending upon the goal of the treatment. These components are:

1. Body Position

Johnson and Saliba were the first to bring the body positioning component in treatment of PNF. The body should be kept in line with the movement. The therapist's shoulder and pelvis should be in the line of movement. Foot of the anterior leg should be place longitudinally on the movement line and the posterior foot should be placed transversely. Use your body weight for resistance. The therapist's should apply the resistance from the hands and arms should be kept relaxed.

The following things are to be avoided to attain patient's right body position during the treatment:
- Uncontrolled or disturbed direction of movement
- Muscle fatigue after giving the resistance
- Postural pain.

2. Manual Contact

It is used to guide and resist the movement and give tactile stimulation to facilitate any muscle. A good manual contact is important because it does not produce any pain due to grip (e.g. Fig. 27.2—lumbar grip). It also promotes tactile-kinesthetic perception and stimulates muscle's contractile ability. The pressure should be applied from flexed metacapophalangeal (MCP) joint thus it helps in developing the patient feeling of security and confidence.

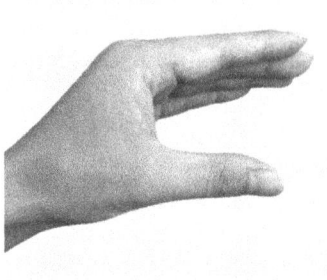

Fig. 27.2: Lumbrical grip.

3. Verbal Commands

It helps the patient in starting of any movement guiding the patient for the intensity of the muscle contraction. The commands should clear, short and effective as it helps the patient in correct movement which is to be produce during the treatment.

Three types of commands:
1. *Preparation commands:* To make the patient ready for action.
2. *Action commands:* To instruct the patient to start the action. It may be *dynamic* or *static*.
3. *Correction commands:* To help the patient correcting or modifying the movement.

4. Vision

It is used to guide the action and give feedback. The patient should look at the movements he/she is doing as it will help in patient control and correct position. Eye-contact can be used for giving instructions.

5. Traction/Approximation

Applying traction or approximation to the joint stimulates the joint receptors. Traction is applied for the elongation of the particular joint/part by stretch reflex whereas approximation is applied for the compression of the joint/part. Traction facilitates movement and thus helps in reducing joint pain. Approximation facilitates weight-bearing muscles in stabilizing activity. The force which is applied should be maintained with resistance throughout the movement.

6. Stretch

Muscle is stretched to elicit stretch reflex. It facilitates muscle contraction and decreases muscle fatigue. A stretch stimulus occurs when the muscle is in fully lengthened position and the maximum facilitation comes from lengthening of all the synergistic muscles. Quick stretch or quick tap may be given on the muscle to elicit stretch reflex.

7. Resistance

The resistance which is to be given should be optimal during the movement should be according to patient's condition and the goal which is required. Resistance during the movement helps in increases muscle strength, motor control and learning. Resistance given by the therapist should be smooth and opposite to the direction of movement. Resistance should not cause undesired symptoms like pain, fatigue, etc.

8. Irradiation and Reinforcement

Resistance to the muscles in an adequate and appropriate intensity and way causes irradiation (spread of response) and reinforcement (to add to make stronger). It is used to strengthen the contralateral limb's muscle if movement of the contralateral limb is not possible. Resistance to a muscle group can cause irradiation and reinforcement to adjacent muscle group working on same pattern, e.g. resistive neck flexion can cause effect on trunk flexion.

9. Timing

The most efficient and co-ordinate movement from distal to proximal is called '*normal timing*'. For specific therapeutic reasons, it is altered by changing the sequence of movement to emphasize a specific muscle or movement which is called '*timing for emphasis*'. It redirects the energy of stronger muscle of prevented movement into the weaker muscles.

It can be done by preventing all motions components of a pattern other than the desired component to be emphasized. It can also be done by resisting the motions components of a pattern isometrically.

10. Patterns

PNF patterns are designed on the basis of functional movements. The motion in PNF pattern is called '*Diagonal (D)*' or '*Spiral*'. It combines movements in all three planes, i.e. sagittal (flexion and extension), coronal/frontal (abduction and adduction) and horizontal (medial and lateral rotation). It should be kept in mind that there should not be undesired trunk movement like rolling or rotation.

PATTERNS OF THE UPPER LIMB (FIGS. 27.3A TO D)

Upper limb include two diagonal patterns that are D_1 and D_2. The above given patterns can be done with or without elbow flexion and extension making following patterns:

- **D_1 Flexion (Fig. 27.4A)**
  - Flexion-adduction-external rotation in elbow extension
  - Flexion-adduction-external rotation with elbow flexion
  - Flexion-adduction-external rotation with elbow extension
- **D_1 Extension (Fig. 27.4B)**
  - Extension-abduction-internal rotation in elbow extension
  - Extension-abduction-internal rotation with elbow flexion
  - Extension-abduction-internal rotation with elbow extension
- **D_2 Flexion (Fig. 27.5A)**
  - Flexion-abduction-external rotation in elbow extension
  - Flexion-abduction-external rotation with elbow flexion
  - Flexion-abduction-external rotation with elbow extension
- **D_2 Extension (Fig. 27.5B)**
  - Extension-adduction-internal rotation in elbow extension
  - Extension-adduction-internal rotation with elbow flexion
  - Extension-adduction-internal rotation with elbow extension

Patient Position

Ideal position is supine lying. Place the patient close to the edge of the plinth.

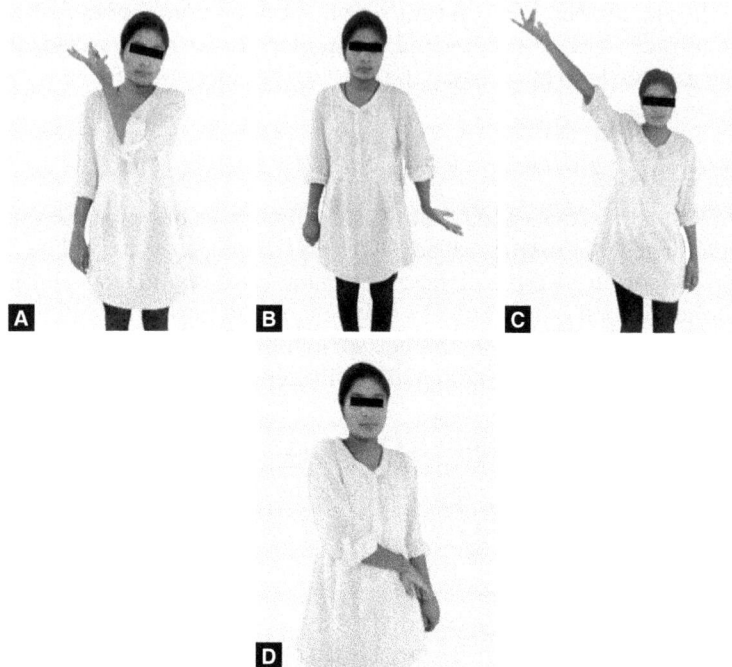

Figs. 27.3A to D: (A) D_1 flexion; (B) D_1 extension; (C) D_2 flexion; (D) D_2 extension.

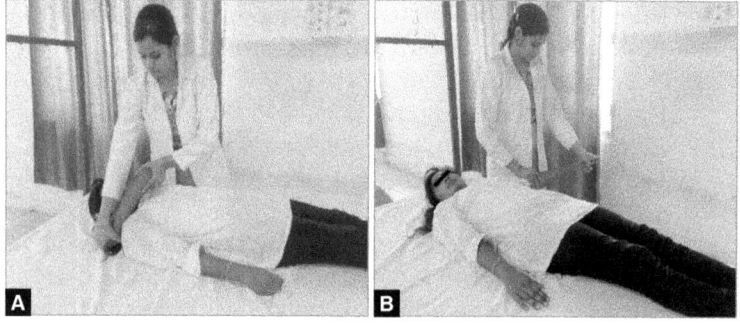

Figs. 27.4A and B: (A) D_1 flexion; (B) D_1 extension (upper limb).

Therapist Position

Therapist stands towards the side of the patient to exercise diagonally in a straight arm pattern.

Proprioceptive Neuromuscular Facilitation

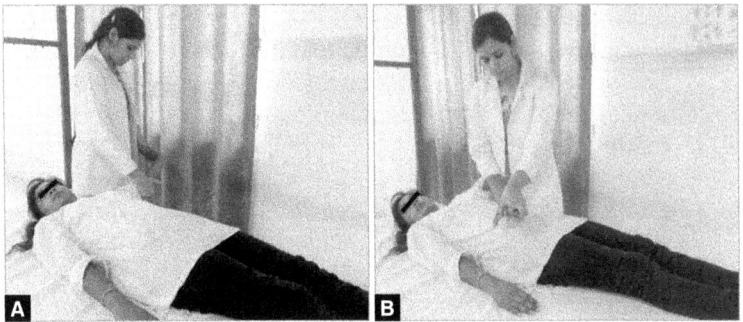

Figs. 27.5A and B: (A) D_2 flexion; (B) D_2 Extension (upper limb).

Indications

- Upper limb patterns help in maintaining normal synergy pattern in patients with stroke and also aids in improving joint range of motion in musculoskeletal disorders.
- Effect of irradiation facilitates the weaker muscles by giving resistance to the stronger muscles.

PATTERNS OF THE LOWER LIMB

Lower limb include two diagonal patterns that are D_1 and D_2. The below given patterns can be done with or without knee flexion and extension with the hip and ankle foot complex in synergy pattern.

- **D_1 Flexion (Fig. 27.6A)**
    - Flexion-adduction-external rotation in knee extension
    - Flexion-adduction-external rotation with knee flexion
    - Flexion-adduction-external rotation with knee extension

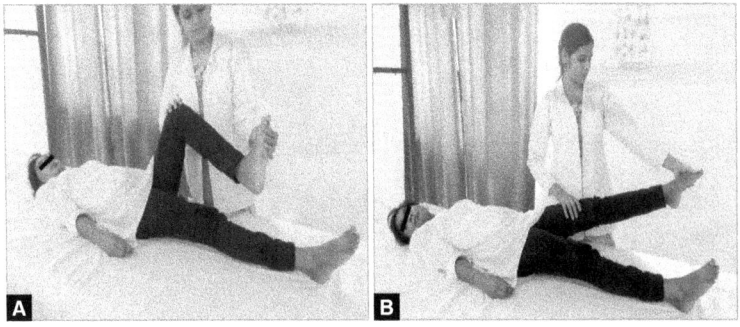

Figs. 27.6A and B: (A) D_1 flexion; (B) D_1 extension (lower limb).

- **D_1 Extension (Fig. 27.6B)**
  - Extension-abduction-internal rotation in knee extension
  - Extension-abduction-internal rotation with knee flexion
  - Extension-abduction-internal rotation with knee extension
- **D_2 Flexion (Fig. 27.7A)**
  - Flexion-abduction-internal rotation in knee extension
  - Flexion-abduction-internal rotation with knee flexion
  - Flexion-abduction-internal rotation with knee extension
- **D_2 Extension (Fig. 27.7B)**
  - Extension-adduction-external rotation in knee extension
  - Extension-adduction-external rotation with knee flexion
  - Extension-adduction-external rotation with knee extension.

Patient Position

Ideal position is supine lying. Place the patient close to the edge of the plinth.

Therapist Position

Therapist stands beside the patient to exercise diagonally in a straight leg pattern.

Indications

- Lower limb patterns can be used in functional activities during rolling on plinth, walking and climbing stairs.
- These patterns also help in improving joint range of motion, incoordination disorders and in lumbopelvic dysfunctions.

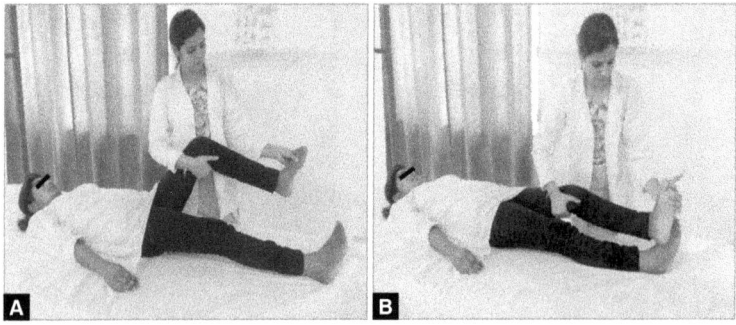

Figs. 27.7A and B: (A) D_2 flexion; (B) D_2 extension (lower limb).

PATTERNS OF THE NECK (FIGS. 27.8A AND B)

Neck patterns include the three motion components that are performed in four pattern combinations:
- Flexion-right lateral flexion-right rotation
- Extension-left lateral flexion-left rotation
- Flexion-left lateral flexion-left rotation
- Extension-right lateral flexion-right rotation

Patient Position
Sitting is the functional position for neck patterns.

Therapist Position
Therapist stands beside the patient to control the diagonal neck motion.

Indications
These patterns are indicated in conditions associated with maintenance of trunk control and stability such as back pain, shoulder neck syndrome, hemiplegia and parkinsonism.

PATTERNS OF THE TRUNK (FIGS. 27.9A AND B)

Trunk patterns include three motion components that are performed in three combinations. The patterns of trunk are as follows:
- Flexion-lateral flexion-rotation (chopping)
    - Flexion-left lateral flexion-left rotation
    - Flexion-right lateral flexion-right rotation

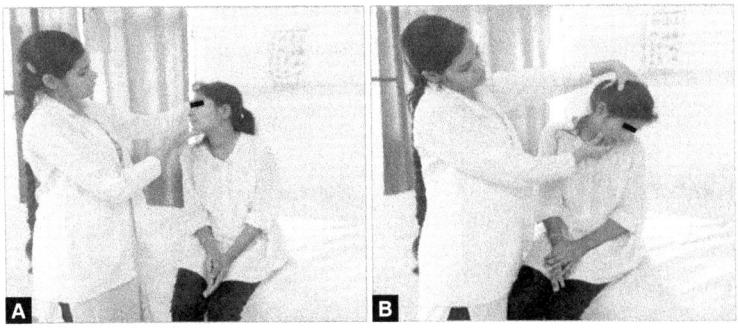

Figs. 27.8A and B: PNF patterns of neck.

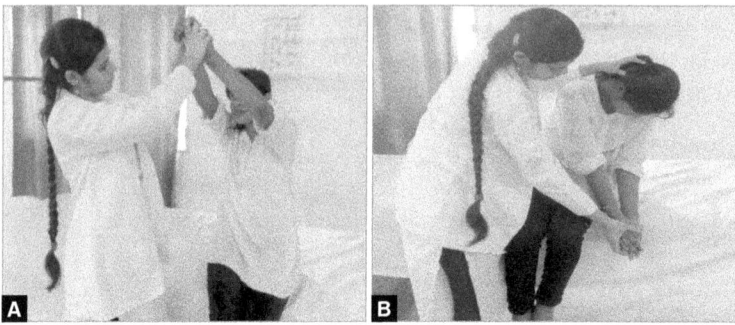

Figs. 27.9A and B: PNF patterns of trunk.

- Extension-lateral flexion-rotation (lifting)
  - Extension-right lateral flexion-right rotation
  - Extension-left lateral flexion-left rotation

Patient Position

It may be supine or sitting depends upon the trunk activity.

Therapist Position

Therapist usually stands beside the patient.

Indications

Trunk patterns help in stabilization of upper and lower extremity and usually implicated in patients with neurological disorders associated with trunk muscles impairment.

PATTERNS OF THE SCAPULA (FIGS. 27.10 TO 27.13)

Scapula patterns occur in two diagonals that are following:
- Anterior elevation-posterior depression
- Anterior depression-posterior elevation.

Patient Position

Ideal position for patient is side lying.

Therapist Position

Therapist stands diagonally either in front or behind the patient or towards the line of treatment of scapula.

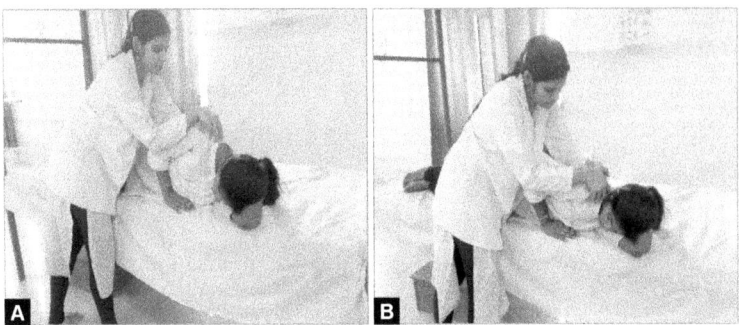

Figs. 27.10A and B: PNF patterns of scapula (anterior elevation).

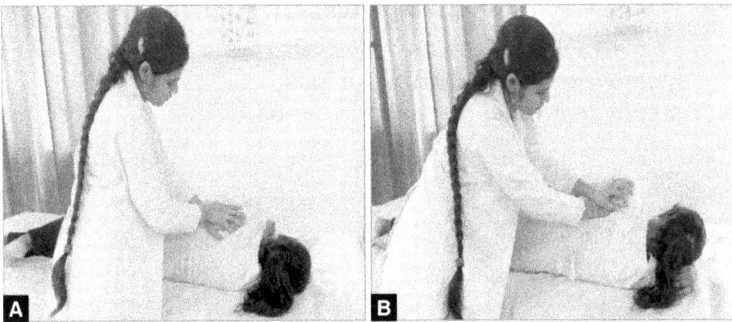

Figs. 27.11A and B: PNF patterns of scapula (posterior depression).

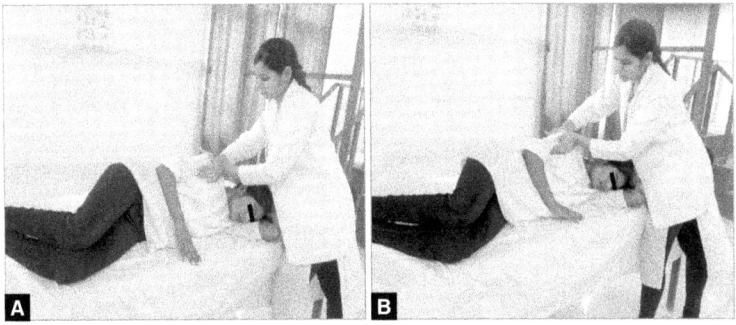

Figs. 27.12A and B: PNF patterns of scapula (anterior depression).

Indications

These patterns help in stability of shoulder and upper back musculature.

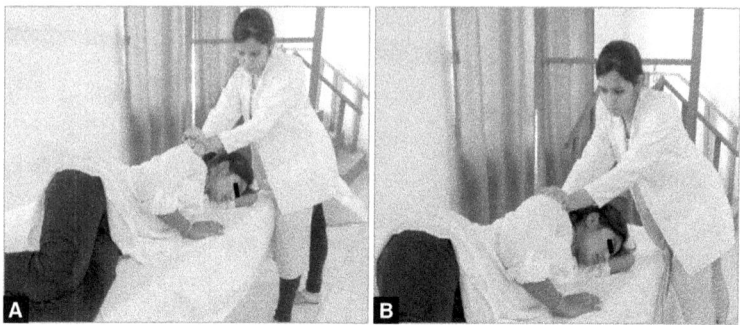

Figs. 27.13A and B: PNF patterns of scapula (posterior elevation).

PATTERNS OF THE PELVIS (FIGS. 27.14 TO 27.17)

Pelvis patterns occurs in two diagonals that are following:
- Anterior elevation-posterior depression
- Anterior depression-posterior elevation.

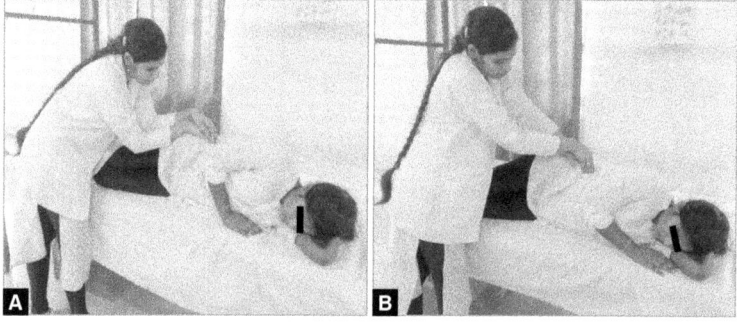

Figs. 27.14A and B: PNF patterns of pelvis (anterior elevation).

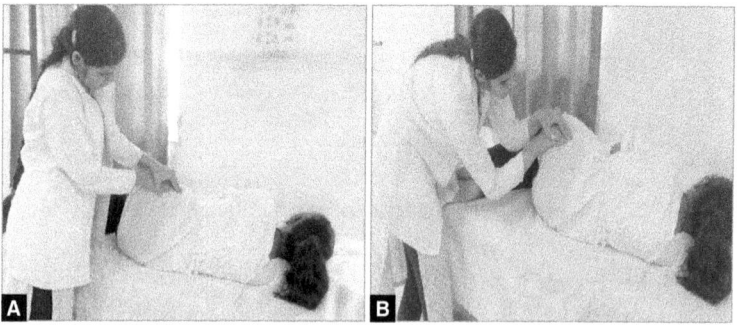

Figs. 27.15A and B: PNF patterns of pelvis (posterior depression).

Proprioceptive Neuromuscular Facilitation

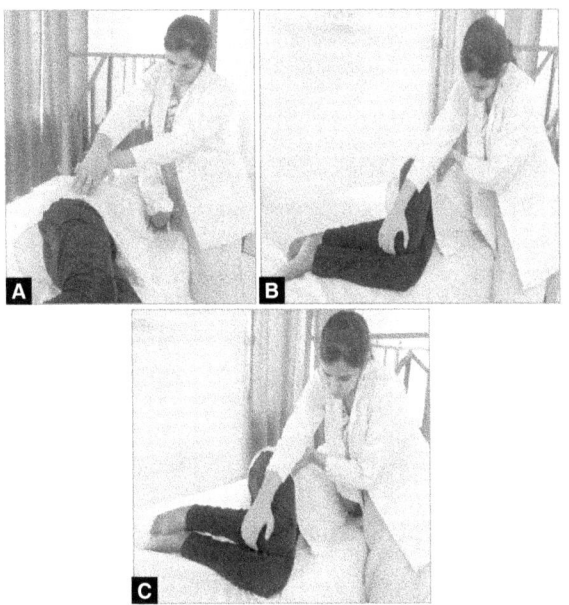

Figs. 27.16A to C: PNF patterns of pelvis (anterior depression).

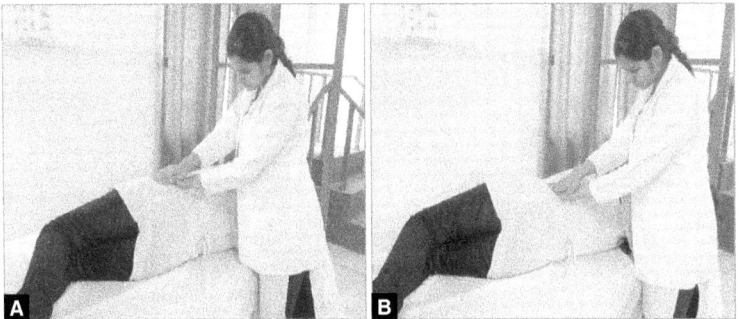

Figs. 27.17A and B: PNF patterns of pelvis (posterior elevation).

Patient Position
Ideal position for patient is side lying.

Therapist Position
Therapist stands diagonally either in front or behind the patient or towards the line of treatment of pelvis.

Indications

Pelvic patterns help in facilitating weight bearing muscles of lower extremity.

PATTERN COMBINATIONS (FIGS. 27.18A TO D)

The patterns of one limb can be combined with the limb of opposite side. Anyhow the combinations may be as follows:

a. **Unilateral:** This is the pattern when only one limb move in pattern, e.g. D_1 flexion of right upper limb.
b. **Bilateral:** These patterns are when two limbs are combined in same or different patterns. These can be classified in 4 groups (see Figs. 27.18A to D).
   i. **Symmetrical:** Both limbs move in same pattern, e.g. D_2 flexion of right and left upper limb.
   ii. **Asymmetrical:** When both limbs move in opposite patterns, e.g. D_2 flexion of right upper limb and D_1 flexion of left upper limb.

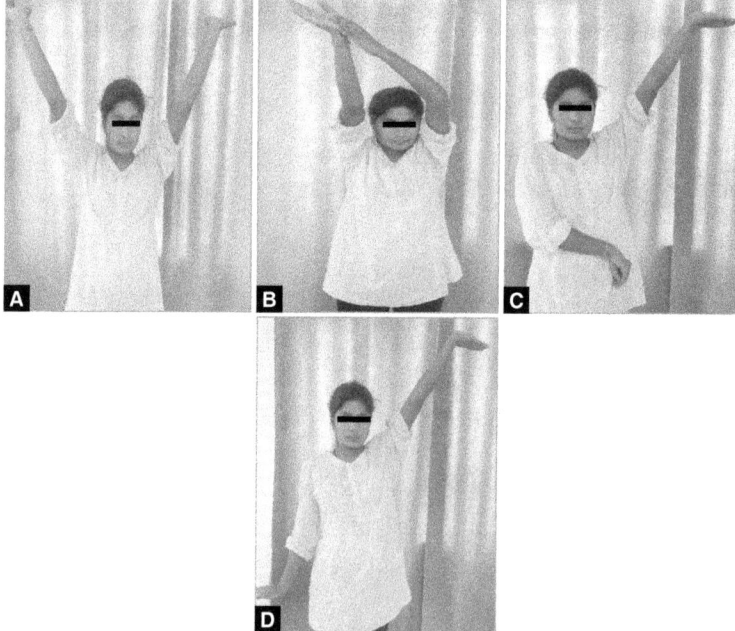

Figs. 27.18A to D: Pattern combinations.

iii. **Symmetrical reciprocal:** When both limbs move in opposite directions of the same pattern, e.g. D_2 flexion of right upper limb and D_2 extension of left upper limb.
iv. **Asymmetrical reciprocal:** When both limbs move in opposite directions of the opposite pattern, e.g. D_2 flexion of right upper limb and D_1 extension of left upper limb.

Facial PNF

The main aim of the facial PNF is to improve the symmetry of face by reinforcing or facilitating the weaker facial muscles. Techniques such as rhythmic initiation, replication and relaxation are useful for the treatment of facial muscles.

Principles of Facial PNF
- The primary goal is to exercise the facial muscles in daily functional activities like smiling, clenching teeth, surprised look, frowning, sucking, blowing balloon, etc.
- Facial muscle exercise should be practiced in a diagonal pattern.
- Facial muscles should be treated bilaterally so that the stronger side can reinforce the weaker side motion.
- Facial muscles should be exercised against gravity. Mirror can be used for feedback to control the facial movements.

Facilitation of Facial Muscles

Frontalis Muscle (Figs. 27.19A and B)
- Therapist instruction to patient: Wrinkle your forehead and lift your eyebrows up.
- Patient keep the eye open, therapist apply resistance to the forehead in a caudal and medial direction.

Orbicularis Oculi (Figs. 27.20A and B)
- Therapist Instruction to patient: Try to close your eyes
- Therapist applies firm diagonal resistance to the eyelids.

Levator Palpebrae Superioris (Figs. 27.21A and B)
- Therapist instruction to patient: Open your eyes and look upwards.
- Therapist gives resistance to eyebrow elevation and reinforces the action.

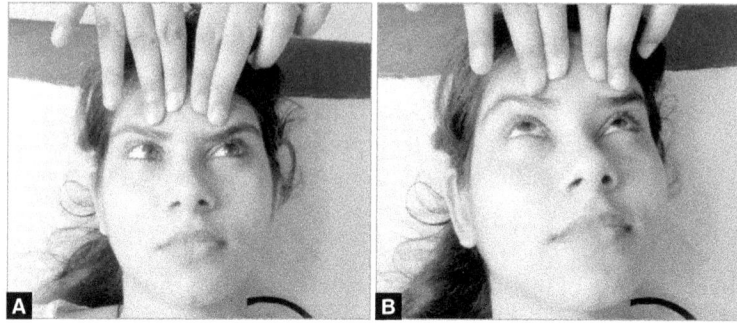

Figs. 27.19A and B: Facilitation of frontalis muscle.

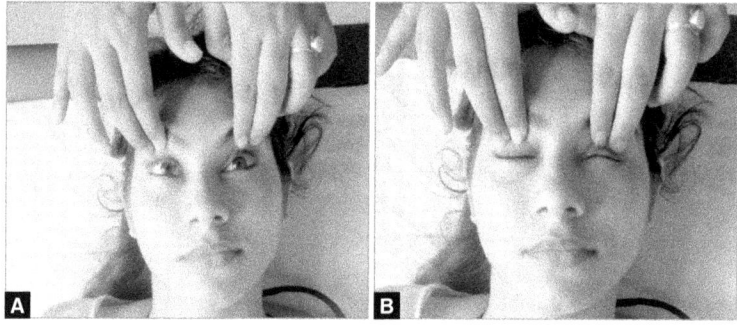

Figs. 27.20A and B: Facilitation of orbicularis oculi.

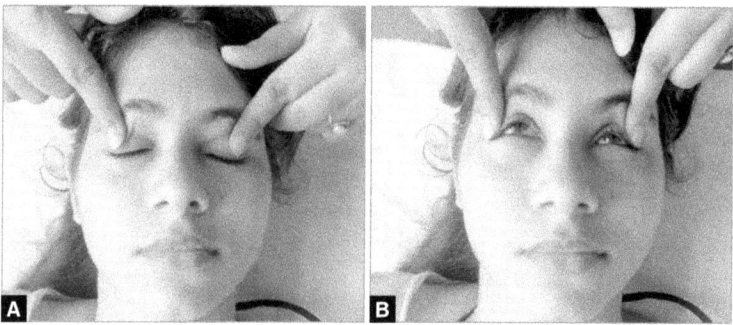

Figs. 27.21A and B: Facilitation of levator palpebrae superioris.

Procerus Muscle (Figs. 27.22A and B)
- Therapist instruction to patient: Wrinkle your nose as you feeling bad smell.

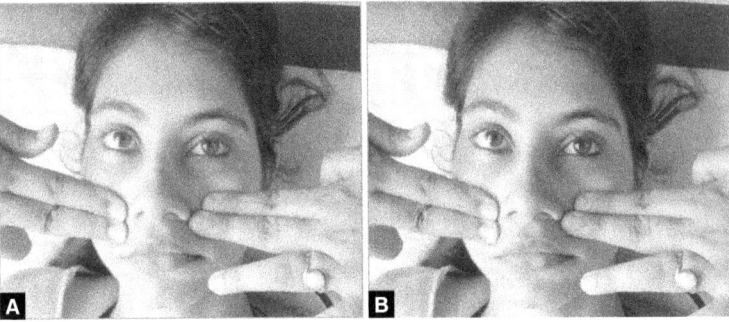

Figs. 27.22A and B: Facilitation of procerus.

- Therapist applies resistance adjacent to nose diagonally downward and outward.

Orbicularis Oris Muscle (Figs. 27.23A and B)
- Therapist Instruction to patient: Purse your lips as if you whistle.
- Therapist gives resistance laterally and upward to the upper lip and laterally and downward to the lower lip.

Risorius and Zygomaticus Muscle (Figs. 27.24A and B)
- Therapist instruction to patient: Smile
- Therapist applies resistance to the corners of the mouth medially and caudally.

Mentalis Muscle (Figs. 27.25A and B)
- Therapist instruction to patient: Wrinkle your chin
- Therapist applies resistance downwards and outwards.

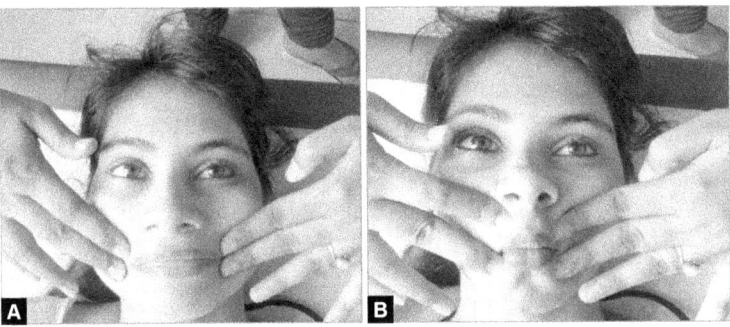

Figs. 27.23A and B: Facilitation of orbicularis oris.

166 Advanced Techniques in Physiotherapy and Occupational Therapy

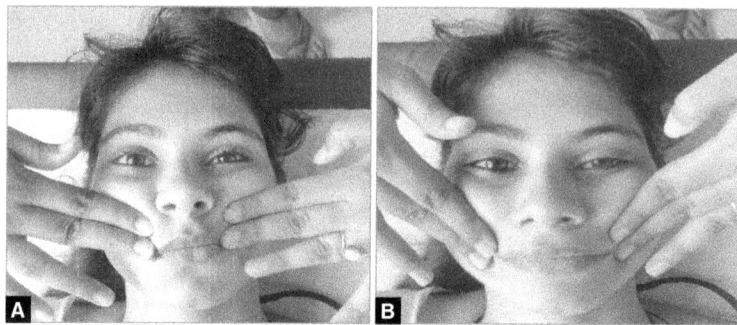

Figs. 27.24A and B: Facilitation of risorius and zygomaticus.

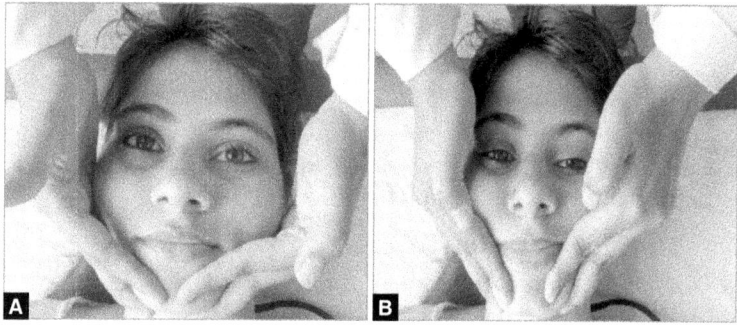

Figs. 27.25A and B: Facilitation of mentalis.

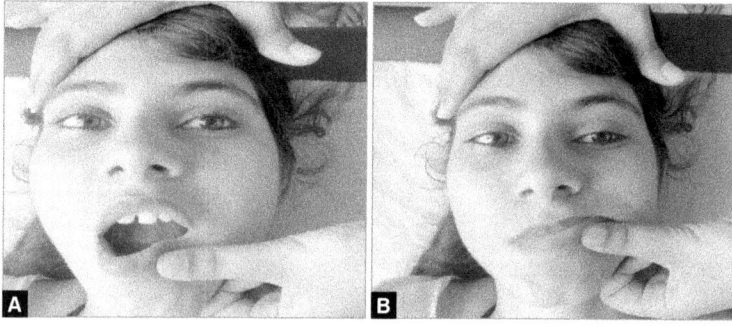

Figs. 27.26A and B: Facilitation of: (A) Masseter; (B) Temporalis.

Masseter Temporalis Muscle (Figs. 27.26A and B)

- Therapist instruction to patient: Close your mouth as if you bite
- Therapist apply resistance to lower jaw diagonally downward to the right and then to the left.

Proprioceptive Neuromuscular Facilitation

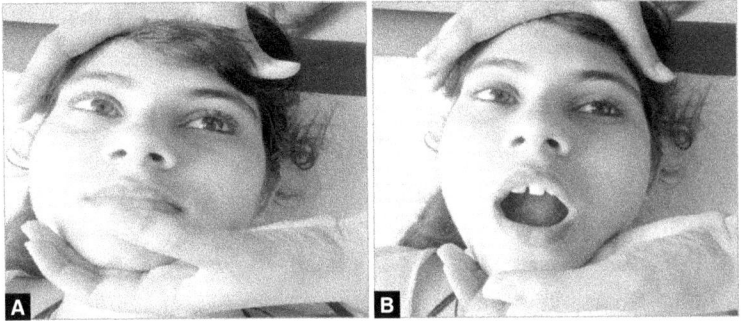

Figs. 27.27A and B: Facilitation of: (A) Infrahyoid; (B) Suprahyoid.

Infrahyoid and Suprahyoid Muscle (Figs. 27.27A and B)
- Therapist Instruction to patient: Open your mouth
- Therapist applies resistance under chin diagonally downwards and medially.

TECHNIQUES

There are various techniques of PNF but the most common and frequently used techniques are:

Rhythmic Initiation

It is rhythmic movement through a pre-decided range. It is started as passive movement and is farther progressed to resisted movement. At the end of the technique the patient is used to do the movement independently. It facilitates the movement initiation, brings the speed of movement to normal, and improves coordination. It is used in the cases of bradykinesia, difficult movement initiation, rapid movement, ataxia, rigidity, and abnormal muscle tone.

Steps for Execution

Step 1: Move the body segment passively in the desired direction.

Step 2: Passively bring the segment back in starting position in rhythm.

Step 3: Repeat the step No. 1 and 2 two times until the patient relaxes and move easily.

Step 4: Increase control of the movement in desired direction actively in rhythm.

Step 5: Now bring the segment in starting position passively in rhythm.

Step 6: Repeat the step No. 4 and 5 two times until the patient relaxes and move easily.

Step 7: Tell the patient to do the movement against resistance.

Step 8: Now again bring the segment in starting position passively in rhythm.

Step 9: Repeat the step No. 7 and 8 until the patient moves easily.

Step 10: Now tell the patient to do the movement independently.

Combination of Isotonic

In this technique, the combination of concentric, eccentric and isometric contraction is given to a muscle group without relaxation. It increases active and eccentric control of movement, coordination, active ROM, muscle strength and power. It is used in the cases of mild ataxia; decrease active and eccentric control of movement, and decrease active ROM.

Steps for Execution

Step 1: Ask the patient to do the concentric movement against resistance.

Step 2: Tell the patient at the end of movement to do isometric contraction in that position.

Step 3: Now ask the patient to bring the segment in the starting position with eccentric contraction.

Reversal of Antagonist

It includes three techniques:
a. Dynamic reversal
b. Stabilizing reversal
c. Rhythmic stabilizing

Dynamic Reversal (Figs. 27.28A and B)

It is resistive movement from agonist direction to antagonist direction without any relaxation. It is started with stronger agonist pattern and ended with weaker antagonist. It increases muscle strength and endurance, active ROM, coordination; and to decrease fatigue and muscle tone.

Proprioceptive Neuromuscular Facilitation

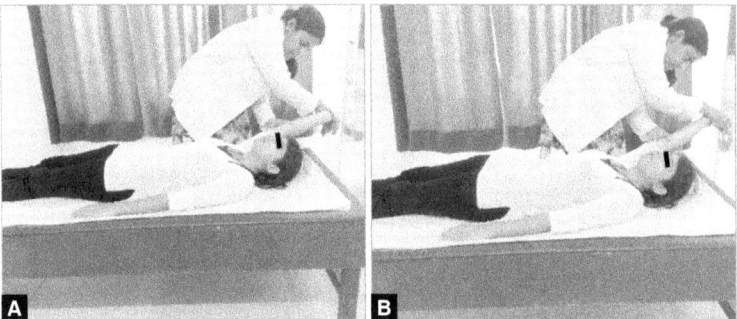

Figs. 27.28A and B: Dynamic reversal of arm.

It is used in the cases of mild ataxia, muscle weakness, decreased active ROM, fatigue and spasticity.

Steps for Execution

Step 1: Ask the patient to move the limb in desired direction (agonist) against resistance.

Step 2: Reverse the distal grip at that time when the range is about to finish and give preparatory command for changing the direction.

Step 3: Give the action command at that time when the movement is finished.

Step 4: When the patient starts to move the limb in opposite direction (antagonist), reverse the proximal grip too.

Stabilizing Reversal (Figs. 27.29A and B)

It is the techniques in which strong resistance is given alternatively to both agonist antagonist muscle group to produce isotonic contraction with very little movement. It is started in the stronger direction. Traction and approximation is used to increase stability. It increases muscle strength, stability, and balance by increasing coordination between agonist and antagonist.

It is used in the cases of muscle weakness and balance problem.

Steps for Execution

Step 1: Ask the patient to do the movement in desired direction against resistance with traction or approximation.

Step 2: When the patient fully resist, move one hand to the opposite side and start giving resistance in opposite direction.

Step 3: When this is done, use another hand to apply resistance to a new direction.

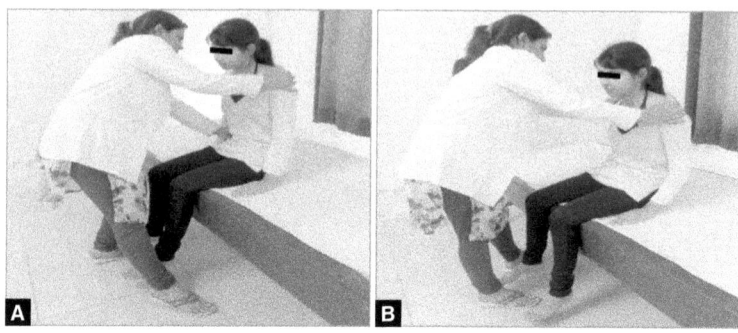

Figs. 27.29A and B: Stabilizing reversal for the trunk: (A) One hand stabilize the upper trunk while other hand stabilizes the pelvis; (B) Both hand stabilizes the upper trunk.

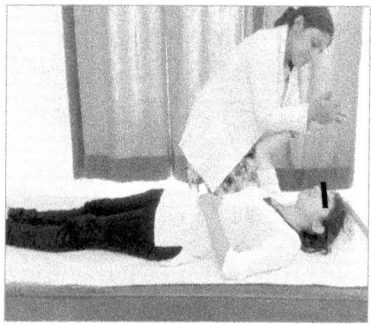

Fig. 27.30: Rhythmic stabilization of shoulder.

Rhythmic Stabilization (Fig. 27.30)

It is a technique where alternating isometric contractions are used. It reduce pain; increase strength, ROM and balance.

It is used in the cases of decreased ROM, joint instability, antagonistic muscle weakness, pain during movement and balance problem.

Steps for Execution

Step 1: Give the resistance for isometric contraction of the agonist muscle group and increase the resistance slowly until the patient builds a matching force.

Step 2: Once the patient responds fully, apply resistance for isometric contraction of the antagonist muscle with another hand without any rest interval and increase the resistance in the same previous way.

Step 3: Once the patient responds fully, apply resistance for isometric contraction of the agonist muscle again with the first hand without any rest interval and increase the resistance in the same previous way.

Note: Traction or approximation is used according to the patient's condition.

Repeated Stretch (Repeated Contractions)

In this technique, the stretch reflex elicited from muscles is used. It facilitates the initiation and range of motion (ROM), increase strength, prevent or reduce fatigue, and guide the motion.

It is used in the cases of muscle weakness, fatigue, inability to initiate motion, and decreased awareness of motion.

Steps for Execution

Step 1: Give a quick "tap" to stretch the muscles to evoke the stretch reflex.

Step 2: Resist the contraction.

Contract-relax

In this technique the resisted isotonic contraction of the antagonist (shortened or restricting) muscles is followed by relaxation and movement into the increased range. It increases passive ROM.

It is used in the cases of decreased P-ROM.

Steps for Execution

Step 1: Moves the joint to the end of the P-ROM.

Step 2: Asks the patient to do a strong isotonic contraction of the antagonist (restricting) muscle and hold it for at least 5 seconds.

Step 3: Now tells the patient to relax.

Step 4: Now reposition the joint to the end of the newly gained P-ROM.

Step 5: Repeat this step until you gain some range.

Hold-relax (Figs. 27.31A and B)

In this technique the resisted isometric contraction of the antagonist muscles is followed by relaxation and movement into the increased range. It increase P-ROM and reduces pain.

It is used in the cases of decreased P-ROM and pain.

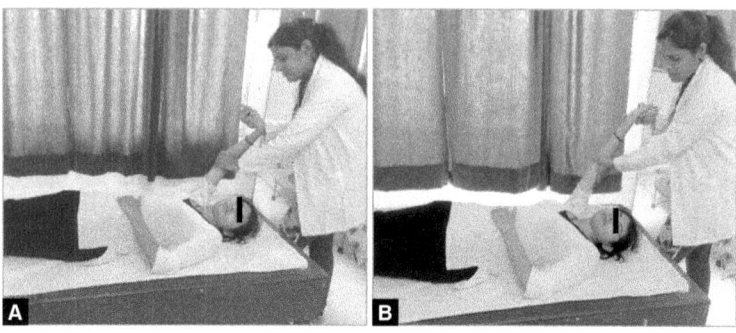

Figs. 27.31A and B: Hold relax or contract relax: (A) Direct treatment; (B) Indirect treatment.

Steps for Execution

Step 1: Moves the joint to the end of the P-ROM or pain free ROM.

Step 2: Asks the patient to do a strong isometric contraction of the antagonist (restricting) muscle and hold it for at least 5 seconds.

Step 3: Now increase the resistance slowly until the patient builds a matching force and hold it for some time.

Step 3: Now tells the patient to relax.

Step 4: Now reposition the joint to the end of the newly gained P-ROM.

Step 5: Repeat this step until you gain some range.

CHAPTER 28

Neurokinetic Therapy™

Krishna N Sharma

Neurokinetic therapy (NKT) was developed in 1985 by a US based manual therapist David Weinstock who has been practicing and teaching manual therapy techniques since 1973 (Fig. 28.1). He cofounded the Institute of Conscious Bodywork in Marin County California in year 1985. He published his first book on NKT— "NeuroKinetic Therapy, an Innovative Approach to Manual Muscle Testing" in 2010.

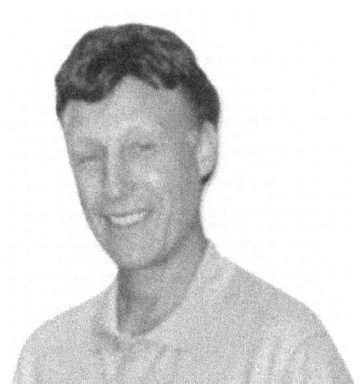

Fig. 28.1: David Weinstock.

THEORATICAL BASIS

NKT is the theoretically based on the motor control theory. *David Weinstock* says, "the motor control centers (MCC) in the cerebellum receives information from the limbic system and then the cerebral cortex before passing the information to the spine and the musculoskeletal system". He believes that the MCC is stimulated by muscle or function failure; on injury, a dysfunctional pattern stores in the MCC which should be re-programmed to treat the dysfunction.

TECHNIQUE

His treatment technique includes application of NKT test on the weaker muscle to stimulate the MCC followed by soft tissue mobilization of the tight muscles for 30-60 seconds. At the end the weaker muscle is re-tested to confirm if the MCC has been reprogrammed.

29 Sensory Integration Therapy

A Sridhar

INTRODUCTION
Sensory integration theory was developed to explain the relationship between the disturbance in interpreting sensation which in from internal and external also and with academic and motor performance. Sensory integration therapy (SIT) is a form of treatment utilizing the various senses of the body which activate the various areas of brain thereby improving the performance of the person. SIT helps to alleviate the absorbing and processing sensory information dysfunction. The input can be given by therapeutic touch or by means of the utilization of the various equipment. The hallmark of sensory integration is applied in context of play, the activity of the children and their reward. SIT is working under the principles of motor learning, adaptive response and purposeful activity.

HISTORY
Dr A Jane Ayres, an occupational therapist first researched and described the theories that are now sensory integration. She had defined sensory integration dysfunction as a sort of "Traffic Jam" in the brain. In 1968, Ayres began calling her theory "Sensory Integration."

POSTULATES OF SENSORY INTEGRATION THEORY
- Learning is dependent on the ability to take in and process sensation from movement and the environment and use it to plan and organize behavior.
- Individuals who have a decreased ability to process sensation also may have difficulty producing appropriate actions, which in turn, may interfere with learning and behavior.
- Enhanced sensation, as a part of meaningful activity that yields an adaptive interaction, improves the ability to process sensation, thereby enhancing learning and behavior.

MECHANISM

In this therapy the participant will be guided in specific activity. The activity is not chosen by the therapist but the environment is created in such a way that participant will be able to choose the activity and therapist will guide the movement. Training the specific activity is not the aim of therapy instead variety of activities will be included in the treatment thereby enable the child to lean the skill efficiently. There are five sensed normally utilized in SIT included vision, touch, hearing, taste, smell but in addition to these, proprioceptive and vestibular inputs are also used in SIT. The brain is the receptor for various senses but impaired brain to some sense have a dysfunction. Physical therapist (PT) can utilize the multimodal input to activate the areas of brain which will reduce the impairments of the patients. 80% of the nervous system deals with processing the sensory input. Out of the above mentioned senses vestibular, proprioceptive and tactile are the fundamental senses. Various form of tactile sensation includes pressure, vibration, movement, temperature, and pain activate tactile receptors. There are two component in tactile sense, one is protective or defensive another one is discriminative system. The SIT is based on the principle of neural plasticity and hierarchial theory of motor control.

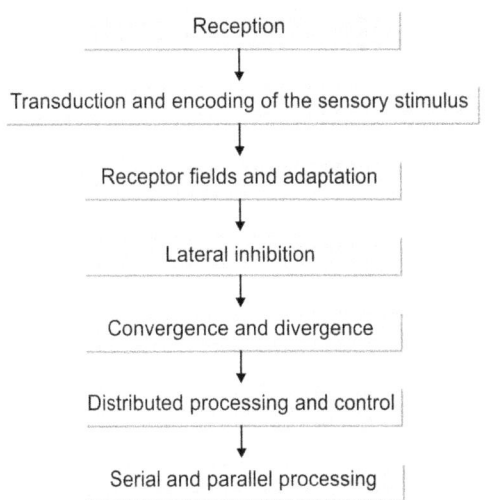

PRINCIPLES

According to Parham, Cohn et al. (2007) the following are listed:
- Intervention should be delivered by the qualified physical therapist or a assistant directed by physical therapist.
- The therapy should be family centered.
- Activities should be rich in sensation.
- Activities promote regulation of affect and alertness and provide the basis for attending to salient learning opportunities.
- Safe environment should be there before applying SIT.
- Activity promote praxis, including organization of activities and self in time and pace.

LEVELS OF SENSORY INTEGRATION

Level 1: Primary Sensory System
- Tactile sense
- Vestibular sense
- Proprioceptive sense
- Visual and auditory senses.

Level 2: Perceptual Motor Foundations
1. Body percept
2. Bilateral coordination
3. Lateralization
4. Motor planning.

Level 3: Perceptual Motor Skills
- Auditory perception
- Visual perception
- Eye-hand coordination
- Visual motor integration
- Purposeful activity.

Level 4: Academic Readiness
- Academic skills
- Complex motor skills
- Regulation of attention
- Organized behavior

- Specialization of body and brain
- Visualization
- Self-esteem and self-control.

MATERIALS USED

- Swings
- Swiss ball
- Slides
- Stairs
- Ramps
- Ball pits
- Flashing light
- Rocking chair
- Cassette tape recorder.

INDICATIONS

- Learning disability
- Developmental delay
- Sensory integration disorder
- Autism spectrum disorders (ASD)
- Sensory processing disorder (SPD)
- Cerebral palsy (CP)
- Speech disturbances
- Lack of coordination
- Gait dysfunction
- Fetal alcohol syndrome
- Neurotransmitter disease
- Modulation disorders
    - Sensory defensiveness
    - Gravitational insecurity
    - Aversive response to movement
    - Under-responsiveness.

SAMPLE ACTIVITIES
Tactile Activities

- Oral activities—licking, blowing, whistles
- Mixing the dough
- Box play

- Dress up
- Applying blanket, sheets, towels pillows.

Vestibular Activities
- Rolling
- Swinging
- Spinning
- Sliding
- Gait activity in unstable surfaces
- Rhythmic rocking
- Swiss ball activity
- Running
- Stairs up and down
- Tunnel walk.

Proprioceptive Activities
- Carrying heavy loads
- Hanging by arms
- Pillow crashing
- Joint squeeze
- Body squeeze.

TEST TO IDENTIFY THE SENSORY INTEGRATION DEFICIT

1. Sensory integration and praxis test (SIPT)
2. Bruininks Oseretsky test of motor proficiency (BOTMP)
3. Motor assessment battery for children (MABC)
4. Clinical test of sensory interaction with balance (CTSIB)
5. Clinical observation of neuromotor performance (COS)
6. Southern California sensory integration tests (SCSIT)
7. Sensory profile (SP)
8. Evaluation of sensory possessing (ESP)
9. Touch inventory for elementary school-aged children (TIE).

COMBINATION THERAPY

It is essential that other approaches can be added to sensory integration therapy. The following are the commonly applied techniques in practice:

- Developmental therapy
- Sensorimotor
- Behavioral
- Coping theory.

PRECAUTIONS

The flooring of the department should be softer which will prevent injury while administering the SIT. Hurrying the activity need to avoid as it should be self-paced and not influential by the others.

CHAPTER

30 Graded Motor Imagery

Manisha Uttam

Motor imagery can be defined as covert cognitive process of imagining a movement of your own body without actually moving your body. Graded motor imagery (GMI) is a therapeutic strategy targeting the activation of different networks in a graded manner. Graded motor imagery progressively engages the cortical neural networks in order to improve cortical reorganization through neuroplasticity. GMI is a three stage process comprising of left/right discrimination training (implicit motor imagery), and explicit motor imagery (imagined movements) and mirror therapy.

SCIENTIFIC BACKGROUND BEHIND GMI

Graded motor imagery involves the neuromatrix (neurosignature, neurotags) and neuroplasticity. Neuromatrix also called "neuronal circuitry" of the brain. It changes all the time as glial cells and synapses change activity. Neurotag is a cortical representation of the brain and neurosignature is a pattern of activity in the neuromatrix. When a neurotag is activated it produces an output, the output defines the neurotag. Neuroplasticity is a cortical reorganization that occurs during development, regeneration or repeated activity across a synapse. GMI works on the underlying mechanism that neural networks which are normally involved in movement planning and execution are also equally active during perception, perceptual reorganization and imagined movement.

PRINCIPLE OF GRADED MOTOR IMAGERY WITH ITS GRADED EXPOSURE

Graded motor imagery utilizes the principle of graded exposure where a stage-wise stimulus—response interrelationship is achieved through an ongoing training program incorporating the

Graded Motor Imagery

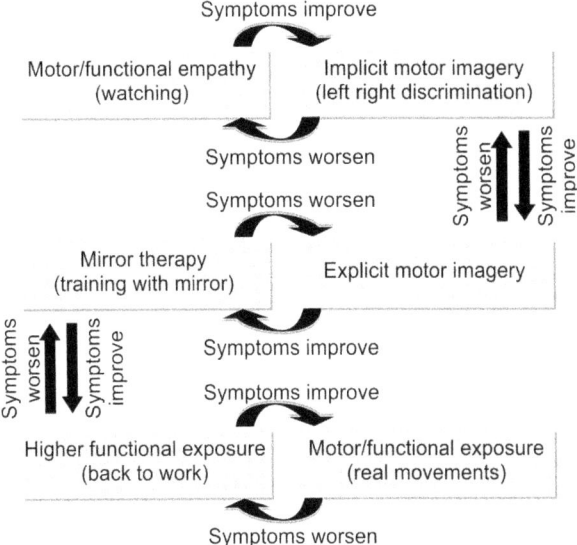

Fig. 30.1: GMI as a part of overall rehabilitation program.
(*Source:* Graded Motor Imagery Handbook)

mechanisms of GMI (Fig. 30.1). There are studies demonstrated that people with complex regional pain syndrome (CRPS) and limb pain can be aggravated by imagined movements. Thus to avoid triggering a pain neurotag that is evoked by imagined movements, a less threatening stimulus is required than imagined movements. This principle is the keystone of physical rehabilitation if an activity is painful or symptoms get worsen then deconstruct it slightly or make it slower or shorter. It should be break into components or reduce the frequency or duration. Left right discrimination is good to start first because of the hypothesized effect of left right judgments to promote intracortical inhibition and therefore the precision of motor neurotags.

Stages of Graded Motor Imagery (Figs. 30.2A to C)

1. Left Right Discrimination (Implicit Motor Imagery) (Fig. 30.2A)
Left right judgment involves two distinct processes. The first is an immediate, spontaneous and unconscious judgment. Second is mental movement by which body part is moving in mind, by using some of the same brain neurotags that are actually use to

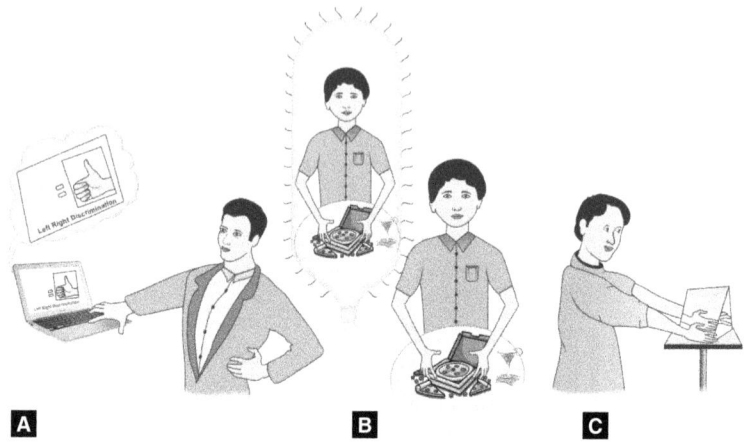

Figs. 30.2A to C: (A) Left right discrimination; (B) Explicit motor imagery; (C) Mirror therapy.
(*Source:* NOI Group Website).

move the body part. Normally, functional representation in terms of body segments exists in the somatosensory and motor cortical homunculi. As a result of this, any sensory or motor stimuli to the part lead to activation of this neurotag. Over a period of time, regional representation group overlapped and altered left right discrimination develops. It activates premotor area which is important in planning of movements and send message to primary motor area.

In this training, photographs of left/right body part are displayed in a variety of postures in front of the patient. There will be less activation of movement areas in the brain during the task. Emphasis will be made on speed and accuracy of performance.

Tools to assess left right discrimination

The best way to test left right discrimination ability is to use the "online recognize program" (www.noigroup.com/recognize). In this, images of body parts are displayed on a computer screen. Body part, number of images, and amount of time on each image is selected on the screen according to the degree of difficulty of image. The program provides a record so that progress can be monitored. Flashcards can also be used which consists of set of 48 cards, having 24 images of a body part and the reverse image including total of 48 images. Changes to response time and accuracy of task can be recorded at the progression of each stage.

Left right discrimination training

Online recognize program software is used for left right discrimination training. Initially, 20 photographs of vanilla hand images can be displayed in a variety of postures on a computer screen for 20 seconds response time. Then response time can be decreased with increase in number of photographs according to the progress of each patient.

Subjects use their index finger to respond which can be made using the left arrow key on keyboard for left sided response and right arrow for right sided response. When a response is made the next image immediately get appear. If the subject not responds, next image will automatically appear when time elapses. Accuracy and speed of response time is measured at the end of each session.

2. Explicit Motor Imagery (Imagined Movements) (Fig. 30.2B)

It is the imagined movement or in the language of neuroscience—the self-generated representation in a brain of a movement without actually performing the movement. There is a small difference in the extent of activation of movement areas in brain such that observing movements cause activation of less movement areas than imagining movements and in turn imagining movements activates less movement areas than the actual movement. Normally, active movements send afferent impulses to the cortex which are programmed and stored in neural engrams. In pathology movements get altered both in quality or quantity, thus leads to altered engrams. In the extent of subjects inability to perform actual movements, observed movements or imagined movements provide a viable alternative. It mainly activates primary motor areas.

It is said that 25% of neurons in brain (mirror neurons) starts firing while observing/imagining movement. It basically relies on observing movement and then imagining the same movement. Emphasis will be made on accuracy but not on speed.

Tools to assess explicit motor imagery

Explicit motor imagery is essentially thinking about moving without actually moving. The main tools required are—knowledge and some basic techniques. Online recognize programme can also be designed for explicit motor imagery by setting up own motor imagery tasks and adjust viewing time and kind of image. Flashcards can be used in the same way as online recognize; they provide movements or postures to imagine. Magazines or photographs are some of other tools that can be used. They may help to imagine moving like someone else.

Explicit motor imagery training

20 pictures of the affected hand in a variety of posture are randomly displayed from the computer screen. Patients are advised to imagine moving their own affected hand to adopt the posture shown in the picture, but the affected hand is resting comfortably, and then asks the patient to imagine returning the hand to its resting position. Stopwatch can be used to record the time of each trial performed. Accuracy is emphasized rather than speed in this trial.

Implicit versus explicit motor imagery

In left right discrimination, if the subject is aware about imagining the movement to confirm initial judgment, then it is explicit motor imagery. To avoid imagining the movement in left right judgment, more practice is required. Brain imaging studies suggest that it takes about 40 judgments, although it varies a lot between people. On the other hand, if the subject mentally moving his limb unknowingly, then it is implicit motor imagery (left right discrimination).

3. Mirror Therapy (Fig. 30.2C)

Mirror therapy is based on visual stimulation. Ramachandran and Rogers Ramachandran were the first to introduce the use of visual illusions created by mirror for treatment of also while watching and observing Phantom limb pain. Mirror therapy works on the mechanism of stimulating mirror neurons in those areas of the brain that have been adversely affected by learned disuse. Mirror neurons were initially discovered in monkeys in 1987 by Rizzolatti et al. Mirror neurons are located in premotor cortex and inferior parietal lobe area of the brain.

In mirror therapy, a mirror is placed inpatient's mid-sagittal plane, thus reflecting the non-paretic side as if it is the affected side. The affected hand will be concealed and emphasis will be on watching the reflection of unaffected hand in the mirror.

Tools to assess mirror therapy

Most important equipment in mirror therapy is good mirror. Mirror box can be made by own or there are commercial mirror box available. Good quality Perspex mirrors should be used rather than glass. The clinician should appropriately train the patient by demonstrating before starting the process. To get the illusion, it is important to make it believable, means taking off jewellery and watch from both affected and unaffected side. The process involves accommodating and accepting the reflection and allowing the brain to be lured into the illusion.

Mirror therapy training
In mirror therapy training, a mirror (30 cm × 30 cm) is placed vertically on a table. The affected hand is concealed (behind the mirror) and unaffected hand in front of the mirror. The practice consists of unaffected side wrist and finger flexion and extension movements and then progress to forearm supination and pronation. Then, ask the patient to try to do the same movements with the affected hand while they are moving the unaffected hand. Increase the speed of the exercise as progress is made.

Evidence for the effect of GMI program
There are many studies that look at the provision of one component of GMI process, but limited research is there looking at the whole process. Moseley made major contribution towards the development of GMI intervention strategy. Moseley report that graded motor imagery program is effective in chronic CRPS1 and conclude that GMI reduce pain by 20 points on numerical pain rating scale in the chronic CRPS1 population. Moseley demonstrate motor imagery reduce pain and disability in patients with complex regional pain syndrome type 1, phantom limb pain and brachial plexus avulsion injury. Lagueux et al. stated that modified GMI seems to be effective to reduce pain and enhance grip strength in patients with nonchronic CRPS-1 of the UE. These results indicate that modified GMI seems to be a promising and effective therapeutic modality to treat this population, which has a high risk of chronicity. Walz et al. utilize GMI in CRPS and demonstrate that after 6 months without further GMI, pain reduced to approximately 50%. Recently, Uttam et al. demonstrate GMI in stroke patients and reported that GMI along with adjunct conventional treatment shows more significant improvement than conventional treatment alone in improving upper limb motor functions and quality of life in patients with stroke.

CHAPTER 31

Postural Drainage

Sudeep Kale

INTRODUCTION

Definition

It is method of mobilization of secretions from one or more lung segments to the central airways by placing the patient in various positions in such a way that gravity assists in drainage of secretions.

Chest physiotherapy is combination of postural drainage (PD) positions, manual technique, voluntary coughing.

The positions are given depending upon the lobes and segments. The positions are given in such a way that the segment of lung becomes vertical to carina, which assist the drainage of secretions towards central airways.

Where postural drainage is used?

- Critical care units
- Inpatient acute care
- Home care
- Outpatient/ambulatory care
- Pulmonary diagnostic (bronchoscopy) laboratory.

GOALS OF POSTURAL DRAINAGE

- Prevent accumulation of secretions in patients who are at risk for pulmonary complication, e.g. conditions which causes increase in sputum production (bronchiectasis, cystic fibrosis, chronic bronchitis). Prolonged bed ridden patients. Postoperative patients and patients on mechanical ventilators.
- Remove already accumulated secretions.

INDICATIONS
- Retained secretions
- Cystic fibrosis
- Bronchiectasis
- Atelectasis
- Mechanical ventilation
- Neonatal respiratory distress syndrome
- Asthma
- Evidence of retained secretions in presence of an artificial airway.

CONTRAINDICATIONS
- Sever hemoptysis
- Untreated conditions like congestive cardiac failure, large pleural effusion, pulmonary embolism, pneumothorax
- Cardiovascular instability, e.g. cardiac arrhythmia, sever hypertension/hypotension, recent myocardial infarction, unstable angina
- Recent neurosurgery and ↑ ICP, i.e. (ICP) >20 mm Hg (avoid head down position)
- Head and neck injury until stabilized
- Active hemorrhage with hemodynamic instability
- Recent spinal surgery (e.g. laminectomy) or acute spinal injury
- Empyema
- Bronchopleural fistula.

BRONCHOPULMONARY SEGMENTS (FIG. 31.1)

Lung Segments	
Right lung (10 segments) (3+2+5)	Left lung (10 segments) (3+2+5)
Right upper lobe (3) • Apical segment • Anterior segment • Posterior segment	**Right upper lobe (3)** • Anterior apical segment • Posterior apical segment • Anterior segment
Right middle lobe (2) • Medial segment • Lateral segment	**Lingula** • Superior lingula • Inferior lingula

Right lower lobe (5)	Left lower lobe (5)
• Anterior segment (anterior basal) • Lateral segment (lateral basal) • Medial segment (medial basal) • Posterior segment (posterior basal) • Superior segment (superior basal)	• Anterior segment (anterior basal) • Lateral segment (lateral basal) • Medial segment (medial basal) • Posterior segment (posterior basal) • Superior segment (superior basal)
Upper Lobe (Right and Left)	
Anterior apical segment	*Picture*
Position: Backward lean sitting in chair, back well supported with pillows or long sitting in semi-fowler's position **Area for percussion:** Under clavicle	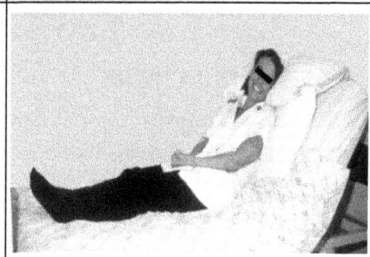
Posterior apical segment	*Picture*
Position: Forward lean sitting in chair, head supported by pillows or head kept on table **Area for percussion:** Above scapula	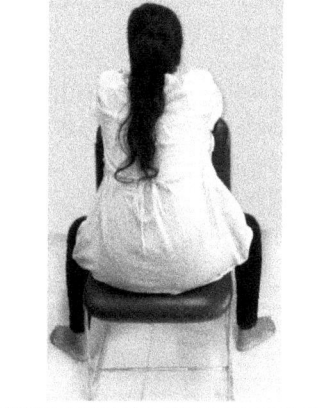
Anterior segment	*Picture*
Position: Supine position, pillows under knees. **Area for percussion:** Just above breast	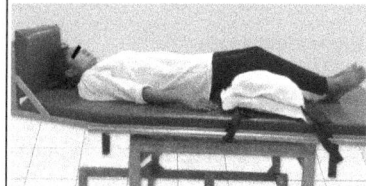

Postural Drainage

Posterior segment (left lung)	Picture
Position: • One quarter turn from prone on right side • Head up position 30–45 degrees **Area for percussion:** Over left scapula	

Posterior segment (right lung)	Picture
Position: One quarter turn from prone on left side **Area for percussion:** Over left scapula	

Right Middle Lobe	
Lateral and medial segment	Picture
Position: • One quarter turn from supine on left side • Head down 15–30° **Area for percussion:** Under right breast	

Lingula (Left Lobe)	
Superior and inferior lingular segment	Picture
Position: • One quarter turn from supine on right side • Head down 15–30° **Area for percussion:** Under left breast	

Lower Lobe (Right and Left)	
Anterior basal segment	Picture
Position: Supine position with head down 30–45° **Area for percussion:** Lower portion of ribs	

Posterior basal segment	*Picture*
Position: Prone position with head down 30–45° **Area for percussion:** Lower portion of ribs	
Lateral basal (right)	*Picture*
Position: Left side lying position **Area for percussion:** Lower lateral ribs	
Lateral basal (left)	*Picture*
Position: Left side lying position **Area for percussion:** Lower lateral ribs	
Superior segment	*Picture*
Position: Left side lying position **Area for percussion:** Below scapula	

TECHNIQUES USED ALONG WITH POSTURAL DRAINAGE

Following techniques are used along with postural drainage in order to enhance the mucus clearance:
- Percussion
- Vibration
- Shaking

Percussions

It is also called as chest clapping. Percussions are performed with cupped hands with rhythmical alternate striking. The moment is at wrist which is alternately flexed and extended. The fingers and thumb is flexed and adducted (Fig. 31.2). The alternate, rhythmic percussion

Postural Drainage

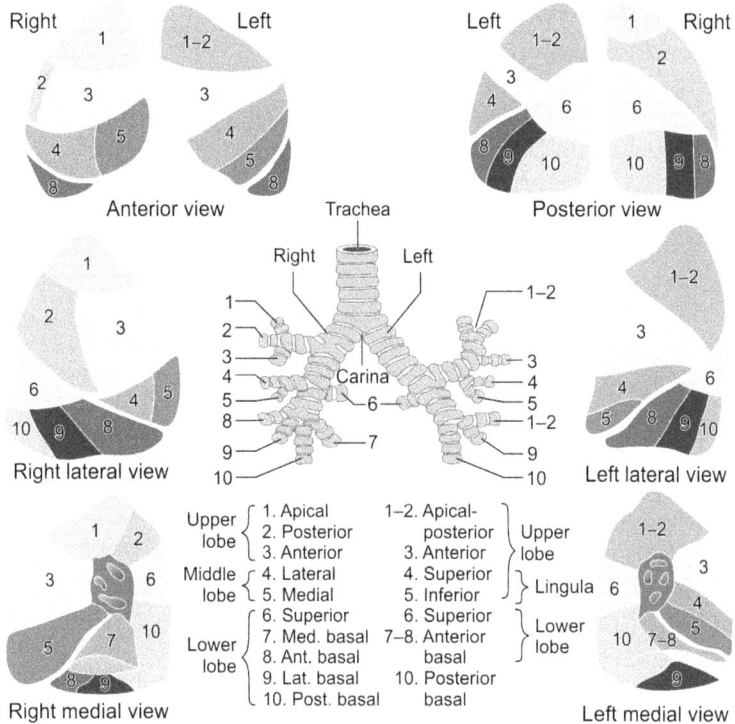

Fig. 31.1: Bronchopulmonary segments.

on chest transmits by the wave of energy. The waves interacts with mucus and causes mechanical dislodgement of viscous mucus. It can be given in both inspiration and expiration.

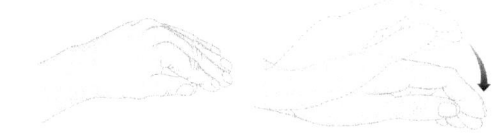

Fig. 31.2: Percussion.

Precautions for Percussion
- Procedure should not be painful/uncomfortable
- Do not percuss on bared skin
- Avoid percussion over breast tissue in females and over bony prominences.

Contraindications for Percussion
- Fractures, osteoporotic bone
- Tumor
- Pulmonary embolus
- Unstable angina
- Chest wall pain, trauma or surgery
- Burns, open wounds, skin infections of the thorax
- Suspected pulmonary tuberculosis
- Lung contusion
- Bronchospasm
- Coagulopathy.

Vibrations

Vibrations are given only during expiration. Hands are kept on chest creating mild compression through the chest wall. Commonly given after percussion maneuver. It creates mechanical waves which interacts with alveoli and causes mechanical dislodgment of secretions. It also increases expiratory flow rate and helps in improving mucus clearance and cough.

Shaking

It is a bouncing maneuver given with hands in which chest is compressed rhythmically. Its given throughout expiration.

GENERAL CONSIDERATION FOR GIVING POSTURAL DRAINAGE

- Never give postural drainage after meals
- Choose appropriate time of day
- Postural drainage early evening helpful
- Frequency depends upon pathology.

Resources Required
- Adjustable bed
- Pillows for supporting patient
- Light towel for covering area of chest during percussion
- Sputum box
- Suction equipment for patients unable to clear secretion (for ICU patient only)

- Gloves and mask for protection
- Stethoscope for auscultation.

Pretreatment Examination
- Auscultate the patient
- Asses the cough
- Look for vitals, Peak expiratory flow rate (PEFR), etc.
- Determine which segments are affected.

Preparation of Patient
- Loosen tight clothing
- Explain treatment procedure to patient
- Teach patient breathing exercises and effective coughing
- Ask patient to cough several times if copious secretions are present
- Adequately hydrate patient
- Humidification is essential if secretions are sticky
- Position patient in correct position
- Make sure patient is comfortable
- Maintain desired position for 5-10 minutes
- Facilitate-relaxed breathing, no hyperventilation/no short of breath
- Apply percussion over desired area
- Encourage patient the sharp, double cough creating adequate expiratory force
- If patients cough is non-productive after 5-10 minutes. Go to other position
- Duration should not >40-45 minutes.

After Treatment Evaluation
- Gradual, slow comeback to normal position
- Look for postural hypotension
- Auscultate the chest: Note changes in breath sounds
- Check vitals.

Positive Outcomes
- Patient removed large amount of secretions
- Change in breath sounds

- ↑/↓ intensity of crepts/crackles/wheez/ronchi
- ↑ air entry
- ↑ O_2 saturation
- Clear chest X-ray
- ↓ dyspnea.

LIMITATIONS OF POSTURAL DRAINAGE
- Airway clearance may be less than optimal in patients with ineffective cough
- Optimal positioning is difficult in critically ill patients.

HOME PROGRAM
- Use pillows, wedges, stack of papers
- Chairs, table
- Explain positions and procedure to family members.

CHAPTER 32

Vestibular Rehabilitation

Dharam P Pandey

DEFINITION

Vestibular rehabilitation therapy (VRT) is an exercise based specialized physiotherapeutic intervention designed to promote central nervous system compensation, adaptation based on neural plasticity and motor learning principles.

VRT can help with a variety of vestibular problems, including benign paroxysmal positional vertigo (BPPV) and the unilateral or bilateral vestibular hypofunction (reduced inner ear function on one or both sides) associated with Meniere's disease, labyrinthitis, and vestibular neuritis. Even individuals with long-term unresolved inner ear disorders get benefit from vestibular rehabilitation. VRT can also help people with an acute or abrupt loss of vestibular function following surgery for vestibular problems. More recently VRT is being practiced in range of central vestibular dysfunctions caused by various neurological disorders.

HISTORY

First initiative for exercise based treatment of vertigo and dizziness was done by Cawthorne Cooksey devised in 1940 are till today commonly used to decrease dizziness. The exercises devised were primarily for unilateral vestibular lesion. Initially, the exercises performed are slow gradually increasing speed as patient tolerates the movement. Since the Cowthorne Cooksey exercises in the management of patients with vertigo and imbalance. Gradually after 2 decade later vestibular rehabilitation therapy started shaping and there numerous number of research evidences exists proving its role in the management of patient with vertigo, dizziness and imbalance. Today vestibular rehabilitation therapy has entered in era where technologically advanced machine based rehabilitation is being gaining popularity such as virtual reality, video game based rehabilitation are few names.

ANATOMY AND PHYSIOLOGY OF NORMAL VESTIBULAR SYSTEM

Normal human vestibular system is made up of three components, a peripheral sensory apparatus, a central processing component that includes vestibular nuclear complex and cerebellum and components on motor output mechanism (Fig. 32.1).

Components of Peripheral Sensory Apparatus

Visual Input

Vision play crucial role in maintaining spatial orientation and thus play significant role in overall balance mechanism.

The oculomotor nucleus proper is comprised of cells that innervate all extraocular eye muscles except the lateral rectus (LR6) and superior oblique (SO4). Remember that it also innervates the levator palpebrae. The EDINGER-WESTPHAL nucleus, which lies dorsal to the oculomotor nucleus proper, contains preganglionic parasympathetic (visceromotor) neurons whose axons end in the ciliary ganglion. Short postganglionic parasympathetic axons then pass from the ciliary ganglion to the sphincter pupillae of the iris and the ciliary muscles of the eye (for changing shape of lens in accommodation).

Vestibulo-ocular reflex play significant role in maintaining balance and equilibrium by stabilizing image on retina.

The nucleus of the oculomotor nerve, considering physiological standpoint, can be subdivided into several smaller groups of cells, each group controlling a particular muscle.

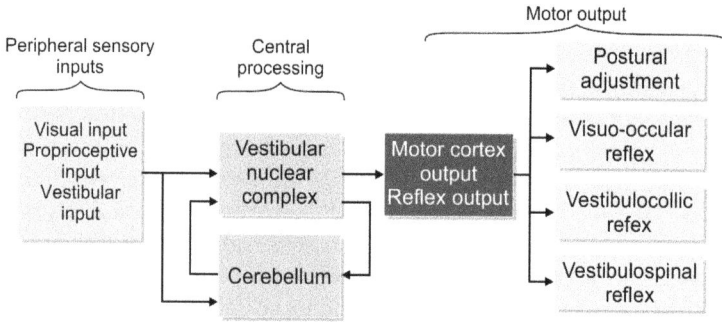

Fig. 32.1: Mechanism of vestibular system function.

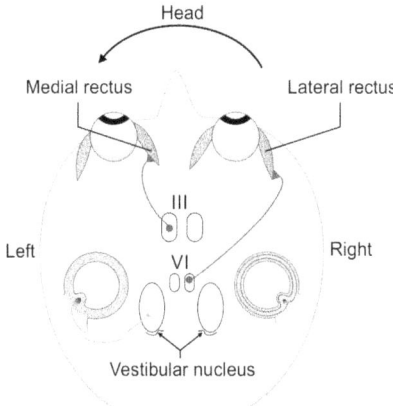

Fig. 32.2: Location of vestibular nucleus.

A nearby nucleus, the Edinger-Westphal nucleus, is responsible for the autonomic functions of the oculomotor nerve, including pupillary constriction and lens accommodation (Fig. 32.2).

Proprioceptive Inputs

There are two way the proprioceptive inputs travels to higher center that is via conscious and unconscious proprioception pathways.

Conscious proprioception is communicated by the posterior column-medial lemniscus pathway to the cerebrum, whereas unconscious proprioception is communicated primarily via the dorsal spinocerebellar tract to the cerebellum.

Peripheral Vestibular Apparatus

Peripheral vestibular apparatus consists of the membranous and bony labyrinths as well as the motion sensors of the vestibular system, the hair cells. The peripheral vestibular system lies within the inner ear, bordered laterally by the air-filled middle ear and medially by temporal bone, it is posterior to the cochlea.

Bony Labyrinth

The bony labyrinth consists of three semicircular canals (SCCs), the cochlea, and a central chamber called the vestibule. The bony labyrinth is filled with perilymphatic fluid, which has a chemistry similar to that of cerebrospinal fluid. Perilymphatic fluid communicates via the cochlear aqueduct with cerebrospinal fluid. Because of this communication, disorders that affect spinal fluid pressure (such as lumbar puncture) can also affect inner ear function.

Anterior Semicircular Canal

The superior semicircular canal (anterior semicircular canal) is a part of the vestibular system and detects rotations of the head in around the lateral axis, or in other words rotation in the sagittal plane. This occurs, for example, when nodding your head.

Horizontal or Lateral Semicircular Canal

The lateral or horizontal canal (external semicircular canal) is the shortest of the three canals. Movement of fluid within this canal corresponds to rotation of the head around a vertical axis (i.e. the neck), or in other words rotation in the transverse plane. This occurs, for example, when you turn your head to the left and right hand sides before crossing a road.

Posterior Semicircular Canal

The posterior semicircular canal is a part of the vestibular system detects rotation of the head around a rostral-caudal (anterior-posterior) axis, or in other words rotation in the coronal plane. This occurs, for example, when you move your head to touch your shoulders, or when doing a cartwheel (Fig. 32.3).

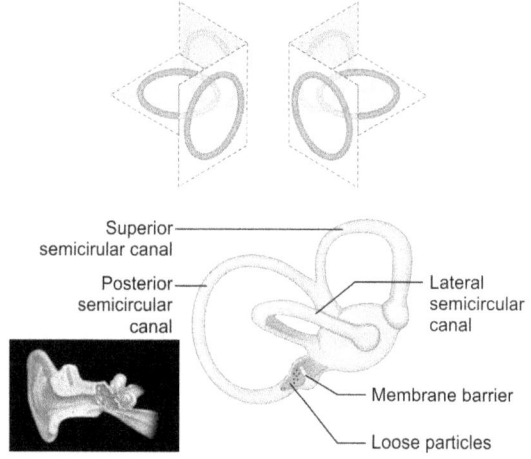

Fig. 32.3: Orientation of the semicircular canals.

Each canal is filled with a fluid called endolymph and contains motion sensors within the fluids. At the base of each canal, the bony region of the canal is enlarged which opens into the utricle and has a dilated sac at one end called the osseous ampullae. Within the ampulla is a mound of hair cells and supporting cells called crista ampullaris. These hair cells have many cytoplasmic projections on the apical surface called stereocilia which are embedded in a gelatinous structure called the cupula. As the head rotates the duct moves but the endolymph lags behind due to inertia. This deflects the cupula and bends the stereocilia within. The bending of these stereocilia alters an electric signal that is transmitted to the brain. Within approximately 25-30 seconds of constant motion, the endolymph catches up to the movement of the duct and the cupula is no longer affected, stopping the sensation of acceleration. The specific gravity of the cupula is comparable to that of the surrounding endolymph. Consequently, the cupula is not displaced by gravity, unlike the otolithic membranes of the utricle and saccule. As with macular hair cells, hair cells of the crista ampullaris will depolarize when the stereocilia deflect towards the kinocilium. Deflection in the opposite direction results in hyperpolarization and inhibition. In the horizontal canal, ampullopetal flow is necessary for hair-cell stimulation, whereas ampullofugal flow is necessary in the anterior and posterior canals.

Vestibule
The vestibule is the central part of the osseous labyrinth, and is situated medial to the tympanic cavity, behind the cochlea, and in front of the semicircular canals. All semicircular canals opens in vestibule.

Membranous Labyrinth

The membranous labyrinth is suspended within the bony labyrinth by perilymphatic fluid and supportive connective tissue. It contains five sensory organs: the membranous portions of the three SCCs and the two otolith organs, the utricle and saccule. Note that one end of each SCC is widened in diameter to form an ampulla.

Understanding various structures and their role is crucial to understand the physiology (Fig. 32.4).

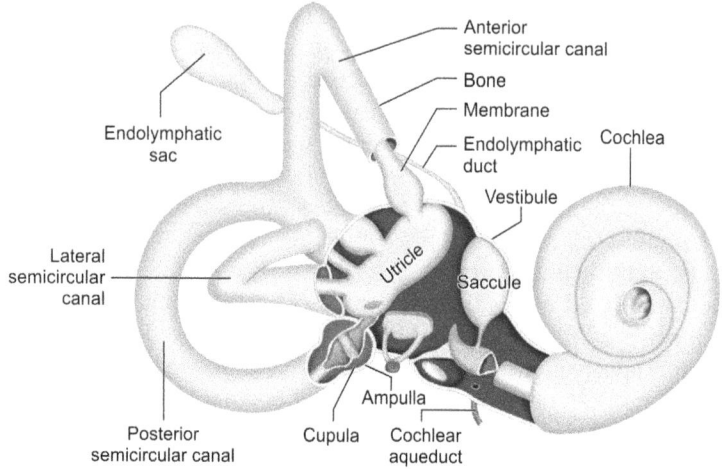

Fig. 32.4: The membranous and bony labyrinths.
(*Source:* Pender D. Practical Otology. Philadelphia, JB Lippincott; 1992)

Saccule

The saccule is a bed of sensory cells situated in the inner ear. The saccule translates head movements into neural impulses which the brain can interpret. The saccule detects linear accelerations and head tilts in the vertical plane. When the head moves vertically, the sensory cells of the saccule are disturbed and the neurons connected to them begin transmitting impulses to the brain. These impulses travel along the vestibular portion of the eighth cranial nerve to the vestibular nuclei in the brainstem.

Utricle

The utricle, or utriculus along with the saccule, is one of the two otolith organs located in the vertebrate inner ear. The utricle and the saccule are parts of the membranous labyrinth located within the vestibule of the bony labyrinth. Utricle detects linear accelerations and head-tilts in the horizontal plane.

Otolithic Membrane

The otolithic membrane is part of the otolith organs in the vestibular system. The otolith organs include the utricle and the saccule. The otolith organs are beds of sensory cells.

Hair Cells

In the inner ear, stereocilia are the mechanosensing organelles of hair cells, which respond to fluid motion in numerous types of animals for various functions, including hearing and balance. They are about 10-50 micrometers in length and share some similar features of microvilli. The hair cells turn the fluid pressure and other mechanical stimuli into electric stimuli via the many microvilli that make up stereocilia rods (Fig. 32.5).

Otoconia

These are calcium carbonate crystals lie on top layer of macula. They are also called otoliths. Otoconia are crystals of calcium carbonate and make the otolithic membrane heavier than the structures and fluids surrounding it.

Macula

The portion of the utricle which is lodged in the recess forms a sort of pouch or sac, the floor and anterior wall of which are thickened, and form the macula of utricle (or utricular macula), which receives the utricular filaments of the vestibulocochlear nerve.

The macula of utricle allows a person to perceive changes in longitudinal acceleration (in horizontal directions only).

The macula consists of three layers.

1. The bottom layer is made of sensory hair cells which are embedded in bottom of a gelatinous layer. Each hair cells consists of 40-70 stereocilia and a kinocilium, which lies in the middle of the stereocilia and is the most important receptor.

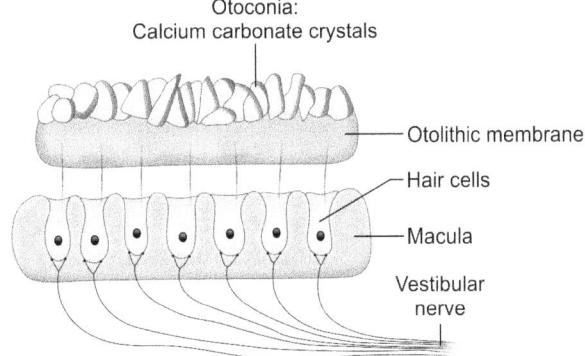

Fig. 32.5: Various otolithic organs in as unit.

2. On top of this layer lie calcium carbonate crystals called otoconia. The otoconias are relatively heavy, providing weight to the membrane as well as inertia. This allows for a greater sense of gravity and motion.
3. The gelatinous layer and the otoconia together are referred to as the otolithic membrane, where the tips of the stereocilia and kinocilium are embedded. When the head is tilted such that gravity pulls on the otoconia the gelatinous layer is pulled in the same direction also causing the sensory hairs to bend.

Ampulla

The bony semicircular canals are situated above and behind the vestibule. These canals are responsible for detecting angular acceleration of the head, they are unequal in length, compressed from side to side, at its attachment of vestibule each semicircular canal dilated these dilatation at one end, called the osseous ampulla, which measures more than twice the diameter of the tube.

Cupula

Within an osseous ampulla there is a crista ampullaris, consisting of a thick gelatinous cap called a cupula. When the head rotates, the endolymph in the canals lags behind due to its inertia and acts on the cupula and many hair cells, which bends the cilia of the hair cells. This stimulation of the hair cells sends the message to the brain that angular acceleration is taking place. They open into the vestibule by five orifices, one of the apertures being common to two of the canals.

Perilymphatic Fluid and Endolymphatic Fluid

The inner ear has two parts: the bony labyrinth and the membranous labyrinth. The membranous labyrinth is contained within the bony labyrinth, and contains a fluid called endolymph. Between the outer wall of the membranous labyrinth and the wall of the bony labyrinth is the perilymphatic space which contains the perilymph. The membranous labyrinth is suspended in the perlymph. The perilymph in the bony labyrinth is continuous with the cerebrospinal fluid of the subarachnoid space via the perilymphatic duct.

CENTRAL PROCESSING OF VESTIBULAR INPUT

There are two main targets for vestibular input from primary afferents: the vestibular nuclear complex and the cerebellum. The vestibular nuclear complex is the primary processor of vestibular input and implements direct, fast connections between incoming afferent information and motor output neurons. The cerebellum is the adaptive processor it monitors vestibular performance and readjusts central vestibular processing if necessary. At both locations, vestibular sensory input is processed in association with somatosensory and visual sensory input.

Vestibular Nucleus

The vestibular nuclear complex consists of four major nuclei (superior, medial, lateral, and descending) and at least seven minor nuclei (Fig. 32.6). This large structure, located primarily within the pons, also extends caudally into the medulla. The superior and medial vestibular nuclei are relays for the VOR. The medial vestibular nucleus is also involved in VSRs and coordinates head and eye

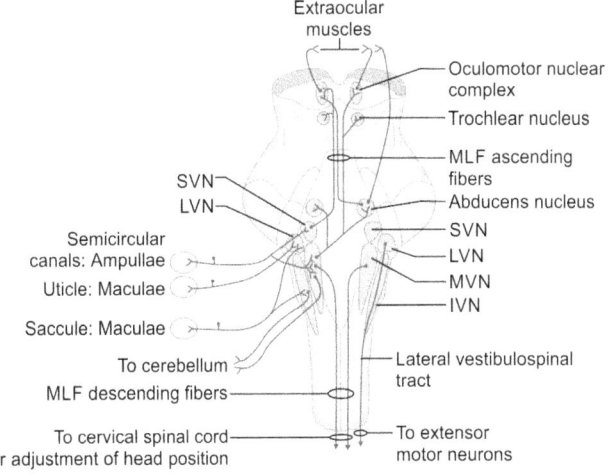

Fig. 32.6: Vestibular nucleus.

(SVN: superior vestibular nucleus; LVN: lateral vestibular nucleus; MLF: medial longitudinal fasciculus; MVN: medial vestibular nucleus; IVN: inferior vestibular nucleus).

movements that occur together. The lateral vestibular nucleus is the principal nucleus for the VSR. The descending nucleus is connected to all of the other nuclei and the cerebellum but has no primary outflow of its own. The vestibular nuclei between the two sides of the brainstem are laced together via a system of commissures that are mutually inhibitory. The commissures allow information to be shared between the two sides of the brainstem and implement the push-pull pairing of canals discussed earlier.

Blood Supply to the Vestibular End Organ

The main blood supply to the vestibular end organs is through the internal auditory (labyrinthine) artery, which usually arises from the anterior cerebellar artery, superior cerebellar artery, or basilar artery. Shortly after entering the inner ear, the labyrinthine artery divides into two branches known as the anterior vestibular artery and the common cochlear artery. The anterior vestibular artery provides the blood supply to most of the utricle, to the superior and horizontal ampullae, and to a small portion of the saccule. The common cochlear artery forms two divisions called the proper cochlear artery and the vestibulocochlear artery. The vestibulocochlear artery divides into a cochlear ramus and a vestibular ramus (also known as the posterior vestibular artery), which provide the blood supply to the posterior ampulla, the major part of the saccule, parts of the body of the utricle, and the horizontal and superior ampullae.

MOTOR OUTPUT: ROLE OF VARIOUS REFLEXES
Tonic Neck Reflex

When the head is rotated in around the up-down axis of the body, there is an increase in the extensor tone on the two limbs on the side of rotation, and a decrease in extension and flexion on the opposite side.

The tonic neck reflex (TNR), by itself, is driven simply by head-on trunk position. As it is not driven by any input related to body stability in space, it does not stabilize the body. However, it is relevant because it combines with the other vestibular reflexes.

The Vestibulospinal Reflex

The purpose of the vestibulospinal reflex (VSR) is to stabilize the body. The VSR is an assemblage of several reflexes named according to the timing (dynamic vs. static or tonic) and sensory input (canal, otolith or both). While terminology varies among authors, the term VSR usually also implies motor output to skeletal muscle below the neck, or in other words, it excludes the neck reflex which is called the vestibulocollic reflex or VCR.

As an example of a vestibulospinal reflex, the sequence of events involved in generating a labyrinthine reflex.

When the head is tilted (rolled) to one side, both the canals and otoliths are stimulated.

The vestibular nerve and vestibular nucleus are activated.

Impulses are transmitted via the lateral and medial vestibulospinal tracts to the spinal cord.

Extensor activity is induced on the side to which the head is inclined, and flexor activity is induced on the opposite side.

When the body is pitched, extensor tone changes according to the position of the head with respect to horizontal. Extensor tone is maximal when the angle of the head is 45 degrees with respect to horizontal (i.e. head is nose up as well as an additional 45 degrees towards upright. Extensor tone is minimal when the head is nose-down and pointing an additional 45 degrees down.

There is also a "righting reflex". When the position of the head or body changes, reflex movements occur that tend to return the head or body to the normal posture. The input to this reflex is vestibular, vision and somatosensation—it is not purely a vestibular reflex.

The Vestibulocollic Reflex

The vestibulocollic reflex (VCR) acts on the neck musculature in order to stabilize the head. Reflex head movement counters the movement sensed by the otoliths or semicircular canals. The neural pathways mediating this reflex are as yet uncertain.

The Cervico-ocular Reflex

The cervico-ocular reflex (COR) consists of eye movements driven by neck proprioceptors. As the COR can supplement the VOR under certain circumstances it becomes relevant when considering recovery from vestibular lesions. Normally, the gain of the COR is very low but the COR is facilitated when the vestibular apparatus is injured.

The Cervicospinal Reflex

The cervicospinal reflex (CSR), also known as the tonic neck reflex (TNR), is defined as changes in limb position driven by neck afferent activity. Analogous to the COR which interacts with the VOR, the CSR can supplement or interfere with the VSR. Two pathways are thought to mediate these reflex signals, an excitatory pathway from the lateral vestibular nucleus and an inhibitory pathway from the medial part of the medullary reticular formation. Their activity leads to extension of the limb on the side to which the chin is pointed and flexion of the limb on the contralateral side. Vestibular receptors influence both of these systems by modulating the firing of medullary neurons in a pattern opposite to that elicited by neck receptors. The interaction between the effects on the body of vestibular and neck inputs tend to cancel one another when the head moves freely on the body so that posture remains stable.

The Cervicocollic Reflex

The cervicocollic reflex (CCR) is a cervical reflex that stabilizes the head on the body. Afferent sensory changes caused by changes in neck position, create opposition to that stretch by reflexive contractions of neck muscles. The reflex was once thought to be primarily a monosynaptic one, however, long-loop influences are now being investigated. Like the COR, the CCR may be facilitated after labyrinthine loss. Cervicocollic reflexes have longer latencies than vestibulocollic reflexes, which gives normal individuals an advantage in head righting over labyrinthine defective subjects.

Somatosensory Reflexes

Other somatosensory mechanisms appear to be involved in postural responses driven by vestibular circuitry as well. It is being documented that somatosensory induced nystagmus interestingly, the subjects with bilateral vestibular loss developed a more pronounced nystagmus than did normal subjects. This implies that subjects with bilateral vestibular loss use somatosensory information to a greater level than controls.

CLASSIFICATION AND CAUSES OF VESTIBULAR/BALANCE DYSFUNCTIONS

Vestibular dysfunctions can be classified in two wide category based of causes:

- Peripheral vestibular dysfunction
  - Due to dysfunction of brain (CNS) UMN lesion
- Central vestibular dysfunction
  - Due to dysfunction of structures other than brain (CNS) UMN lesion

Usually the causes in otogenic origin are considered as true vestibular dysfunctions. But there are various nonotogenic causes results in vestibular and balance impairment these are preferably not considered true vestibular dysfunctions (Table 32.1).

Table 32.1: Otogenic and nonotogenic causes of vestibular dysfunction.

Otogenic causes	Nonotogenic causes
Benign paroxysmal positional vertigo	Degenerative: Age-related decline in balance function
Labyrinthitis	Infectious: Meningitis, encephalitis, epidural abscess, syphilis
Vestibular neuronitis	Circulatory: Cerebral or cerebellar ischemia or hypoperfusion, stroke, lateral medullary syndrome (Wallenberg's syndrome)
Trauma	Structural: Arnold-Chiari malformation, hydrocephalus
Perilymph fistula	Systemic: Multiple sclerosis, Parkinson's disease
Superior canal dehiscence syndrome	Vitamin deficiency: Vitamin B_{12} deficiency neuropathy
Bilateral vestibulopathy	Malignancy: Neoplasms of CNS or posterior fossa
	Other: Mal de debarquement, motion sickness, migraine associated vertigo, toxins, drugs, medications

EXAMINATION AND ASSESSMENT OF PATIENTS WITH VESTIBULAR DYSFUNCTION

Patients with vestibular dysfunction means the patients who have vertigo, dizziness or sense of impaired balance. These patients need to evaluated very carefully specially taking history, a properly taken history would mostly tell examiner an idea about what to examine (Fig. 32.7).

While taking history clinician must look for clue to rule out the symptom whether it is vertigo, light-headedness or impaired

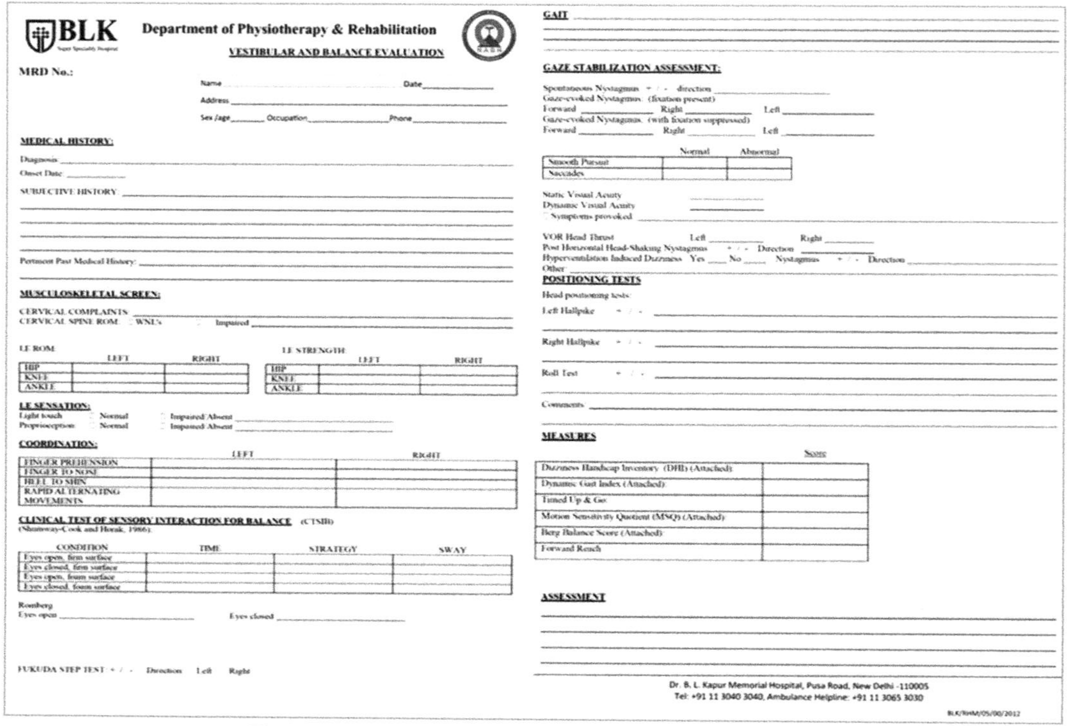

BLK Super Speciality Hospital

Department of Physiotherapy & Rehabilitation

VESTIBULAR AND BALANCE EVALUATION

MRD No.:

Name ____ Date ____

Address ____

Sex /age ____ Occupation ____ Phone ____

MEDICAL HISTORY:

Diagnosis ____

Onset Date ____

SUBJECTIVE HISTORY ____

Pertinent Past Medical History ____

MUSCULOSKELETAL SCREEN:

CERVICAL COMPLAINTS ____

CERVICAL SPINE ROM: WNL's Impaired ____

LE ROM

	LEFT	RIGHT
HIP		
KNEE		
ANKLE		

LE STRENGTH

	LEFT	RIGHT
HIP		
KNEE		
ANKLE		

LE SENSATION:

Light touch Normal Impaired/Absent ____

Proprioception Normal Impaired/Absent ____

COORDINATION:

	LEFT	RIGHT
FINGER PREHENSION		
FINGER TO NOSE		
HEEL TO SHIN		
RAPID ALTERNATING MOVEMENTS		

CLINICAL TEST OF SENSORY INTERACTION FOR BALANCE (CTSIB) (Shumway-Cook and Horak, 1986):

CONDITION	TIME	STRATEGY	SWAY
Eyes open, firm surface			
Eyes closed, firm surface			
Eyes open, foam surface			
Eyes closed, foam surface			

Romberg

Eyes open ____ Eyes closed ____

FUKUDA STEP TEST + / - Direction Left Right

GAIT ____

GAZE STABILIZATION ASSESSMENT:

Spontaneous Nystagmus + / - direction ____

Gaze-evoked Nystagmus (fixation present)

Forward ____ Right ____ Left ____

Gaze-evoked Nystagmus (with fixation suppressed)

Forward ____ Right ____ Left ____

	Normal	Abnormal
Smooth Pursuit		
Saccades		

Static Visual Acuity ____

Dynamic Visual Acuity ____

Symptoms provoked ____

VOR Head Thrust Left ____ Right ____

Post Horizontal Head-Shaking Nystagmus + / - Direction ____

Hyperventilation Induced Dizziness Yes ___ No ___ Nystagmus + / - Direction ____

Other ____

POSITIONING TESTS

Head positioning tests:

Left Hallpike + / - ____

Right Hallpike + / - ____

Roll Test + / - ____

Comments ____

MEASURES

	Score
Dizziness Handicap Inventory (DHI) (Attached)	
Dynamic Gait Index (Attached)	
Timed Up & Go	
Motion Sensitivity Quotient (MSQ) (Attached)	
Berg Balance Score (Attached)	
Forward Reach	

ASSESSMENT

Dr. B. L. Kapur Memorial Hospital, Pusa Road, New Delhi -110005

Tel: +91 11 3040 3040, Ambulance Helpline: +91 11 3065 3030

BLK/RHM/05/00/2012

Fig. 32.7: Sample vestibular assessment form.

balance. Asking questions like *"do you feel like you might pass out,"* are questions which suggest that the patient is describing a feeling of faintness or light-headedness, similarly asking *"does it feel like you're on an amusement ride,"* and *"are you feel spinning* may suggests true vertigo whereas questions like *"does it only happen when you're on your feet"* and *"does it get much better if you touch things"* to screen the impaired balance.

Taking History

A carefully taken history would probably suggests that the patient is either having light-headedness, imbalance or vertigo, based of symptom you may proceed further evaluation.

If you found light-headedness was the principle symptom then carefully look for if there is any associated symptom as it could be because of simple dehydration, orthostatic hypotension, and cardiac arrhythmias especially when it is spontaneous in nature. In this case you may need physician help to diagnose the root cause of symptom.

If the primary symptom is sense of imbalance or unsteadiness then you must look for if the symptom is associated with head motion or its nature is vertiginous, episodic. A vertiginous, episodic symptoms suggest vestibular involvement whereas nonvertiginous, episodic of persistent symptoms suggest CNS involvement.

Once you have carefully taken history you will be able to conclude what set of examination you are going to perform to rule out the origin of the symptom. For example, you may found that patient's problem has root origin from inflammatory nature like labrynthitis or vestibular neuritis you can refer your patient for appropriate management similarly if you found clue that patient problem is originating from CNS than you may plan set of CNS examination testing motor function, cerebellar function.

Before developing any vestibular rehabilitation program it is very important to do system screening you may need to do find principle origin of symptom, it includes examination of cerebellar function. Motor examination, proprioceptive/sensory examination and musculoskeletal screening for muscle strength/deformity, etc.

Based on history you will be able to plan the appropriate system screening and examination of patient, remember the mechanism explained in beginning of this chapter. You need to examine the sensory inputs that is visual, proprioceptive and vestibular that includes examination for benign paroxysmal vertigo, after that you need to examine to rule out if there is problem in central processing, similarly screen if motor components impairment exists. Table 32.2 summarizes various components and related tests.

Table 32.2: Various components and their related tests.

Screening component	Test suggested
Musculoskeletal and motor functions	• Cervical spine examination • Rule out vertebrobasilar insufficiency • Lower limb manual muscle testing and range of motion • Musculoskeletal deformity
Cerebellar functions	• Finger to nose rule out dysmetria • Rapid alternating movements rule out dysdiadochokinesia
Visuo-motor functions	• Smooth pursuit • Saccades
Proprioception	• Rhomberg test • Combined test for sensory motor integration (CTSMI)
Vestibular system	• Head thrust test • Dix-Halpike test • Modified Dix-Halpike test

Specific Test for Benign Paroxysmal Vertigo

Test for Anterior Semicircular Canal (Table 32.3)

Table 32.3: Test for anterior semicircular canal.

Test name	Finding to observe
Dix-Hallpike manuever test	Nystagmus: Duration/Characteristic
	Appearance of symptom that is vertigo

Procedure of Testing (Fig. 32.8)
Start Position
- Long sitting—head turned towards 45° to tested side patient lay down to supine, head extends 30° over the edge of the bed.

Findings to be Observed
- Torsional down beat nystagmus with vertigo.

Note: Torsional down beat nystagmus without vertigo may suggest posterior fossa lesion so we must rule out that too.

Vestibular Rehabilitation

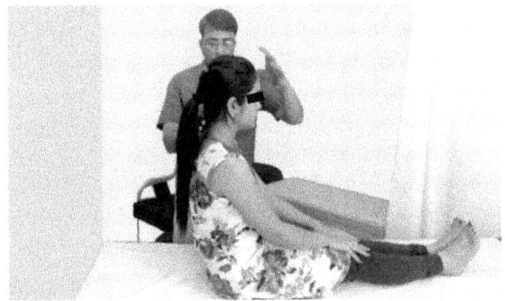

Fig. 32.8: Procedure of testing for anterior semicircular canal.

Test for Posterior Semicircular Canal (Table 32.4)

Table 32.4: Test for posterior semicircular canal.

Test name	Finding to observe
Dix-Hallpike manuever test	Nystagmus: Duration/Characteristic
	Appearance of symptom that is vertigo

Start Position
- Long sitting—head turned towards 45° to tested side patient lay down to supine, head extends 30° over the edge of the bed.

Findings to be Observed
- Torsional upbeating (upper poles of the eyes appear to beat toward the patient's forehead). Nystagmus with vertigo.

Test for Horizontal Semicircular Canal (Table 32.5)

Table 32.5: Test for horizontal semicircular canal.

Test name	Finding to observe
Modified Dix-Hallpike manuever test	Nystagmus: Duration/Characteristic
	Appearance of symptom that is vertigo

Start Position
- Long sitting—patient lay down to supine, head end (may use pillows) elevated 30°, head turned to testing side (Fig. 32.9).

Findings to be Observed
- Horizontal nystagmus with vertigo.

Note: Horizontal nystagmus without vertigo may suggest posterior fossa lesion
- Variation must be observed

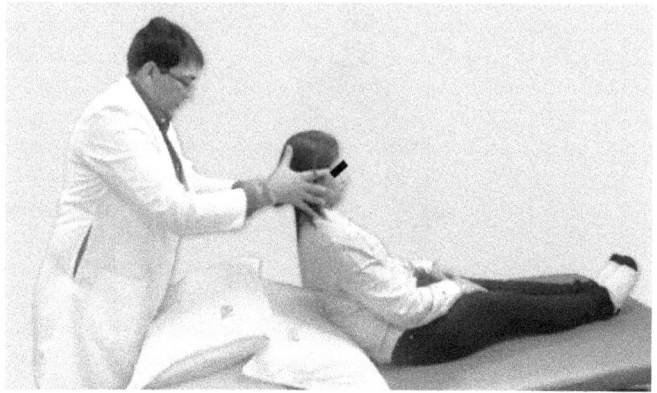

Fig. 32.9: Procedure of testing for horizontal semicircular canal.

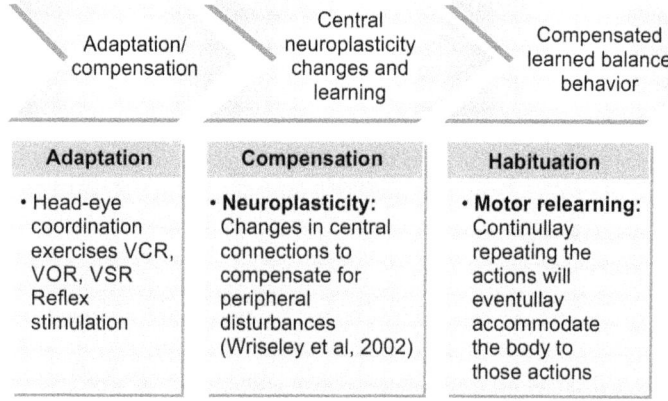

Fig. 32.10: Principles of vestibular rehabilitation therapy.

- Horizontal nystagmus with geotropic pattern suggests canalithiasis
- Horizontal nystagmus with a geotropic pattern suggests cupulolithiasis.

After appropriate history taking and thorough examination you will be able to know the most dysfunctional area of sensory motor system of balance accordingly you can design an effective vestibular rehabilitation plan.

PRINCIPLES OF VESTIBULAR REHABILITATION THERAPY

Principles of vestibular rehabilitation therapy is shown in Figure 32.10.

INDICATIONS OF VESTIBULAR REHABILITATION THERAPY

Indications of vestibular rehabilitation therapy are shown in Table 32.6.

Table 32.6: Indications of vestibular rehabilitation therapy.

Strongly recommended	Specific interventions for benign paroxysmal positional vertigo (BPPV)
	Unilateral loss (e.g. vestibular neuritis or acoustic neuroma)
	Bilateral loss (e.g. gentamicin ototoxicity)
	Meniere's syndrome
	Perilymphatic fistula
	Post-traumatic vertigo
	Multifactorial disequilibrium of the elderly
	Psychogenic vertigo for desensitization
	Phobic postural vertigo
	Interventions for central vertigo (e.g. non-progressive neurological disorders like CVA, head injury associated imbalance/vertigo)
Moderately recommended	Cerebellar degenerations
	Basal ganglia syndromes
	Idiopathic motion intolerance

VESTIBULAR REHABILITATION THERAPY PROGRAM

Vestibular rehabilitation therapy program is set of maneuvers and specifically designed exercises. It can be divided in three category (Table 32.7).

Table 32.7: Categories of vestibular rehabilitation therapy program.

Liberatory maneuvers	Vertigo adaptation exercises	Compensation and habituation exercises
Eplye's maneuver	VOR reflex stimulation exercises	Proprioceptive stimulation exercises
Barbecue role maneuver	Brandt Daroff exercises	Gait exercises
		Combined exercises
		Coordination exercises
		VSR stimulation exercises

Eplye's Maneuver

The Epley maneuver or repositioning maneuver is a maneuver used to treat benign paroxysmal positional vertigo (BPPV) of the posterior or anterior canals. It works by allowing free floating particles from the affected semicircular canal to be relocated, using gravity, back into the utricle, where they can no longer stimulate the cupula, therefore, relieving the patient of bothersome vertigo. It is performed after confirmation of a diagnosis of BPPV using the Dix-Hallpike test and has a reported success rate of between 90% and 95%. This maneuver was developed by Dr John Epley and first described in 1980.

The following sequence of positions describes the Epley maneuver (Fig. 32.11):

The entire procedure may be repeated two more times, for a total of three times.

During every step of this procedure the patient may experience some dizziness (Fig. 32.12).

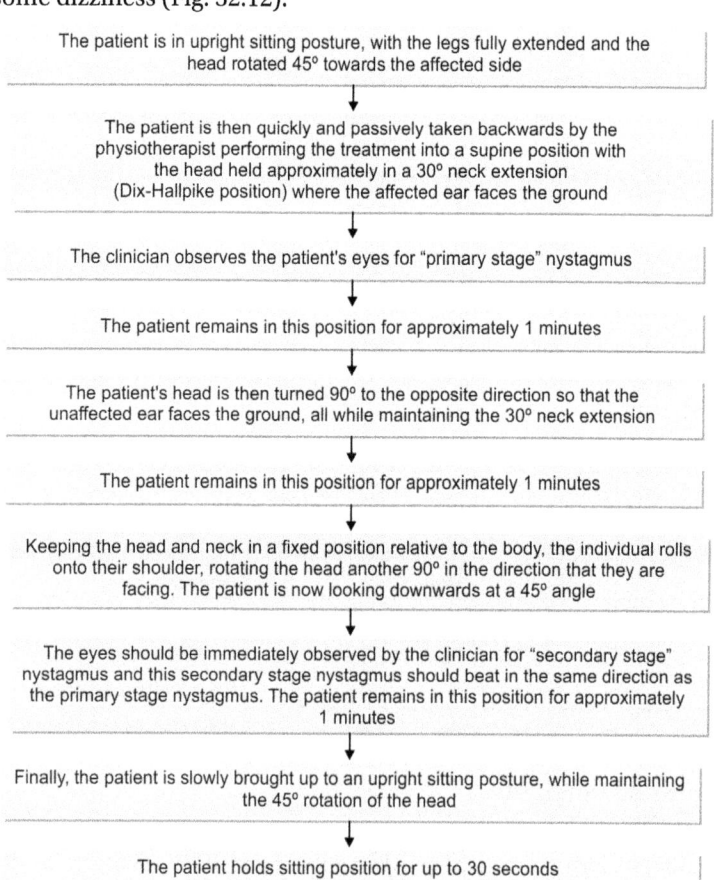

Fig. 32.11: Sequence of positions of Eplye's maneuver.

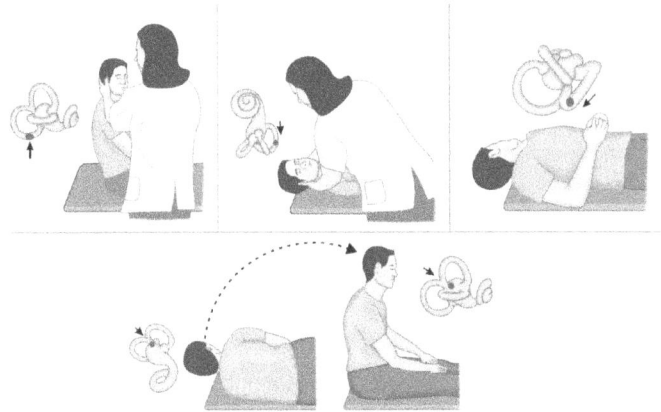

Fig. 32.12: Demonstrating Epley maneuver.

With the patient sitting on a table or flat surface with head turned away from the affected side
↓
Quickly put the patient into the side-lying position, toward the affected side with the head turned up. Nystagmus will occur shortly after arriving at the side-lying position. Keep the patient here until at least 20 seconds after all nystagmus has ceased
↓
Quickly move the patient back up and through the sitting position so that he or she is in the opposite side-lying position with head facing down (head did not turn during the position change). Keep the patient in this position for ~30 seconds (some recommend up to 10 minutes)
↓
At a normal or slow rate, bring the patient back up to the sitting position

Fig. 32.13: Sequence of Semont maneuver.

Semont Liberatory Maneuver

Refer Figures 32.13 and 32.14.

Lempert 360-(Barbeque) Degree Roll Maneuver to Treat Horizontal Canal BPPV

Refer Figures 32.15 and 32.16.

Cawthorne Cooksey Exercises

Cawthorne Cooksey exercises devised in 1940 are till today commonly used to decrease dizziness. The exercises devised were primarily for

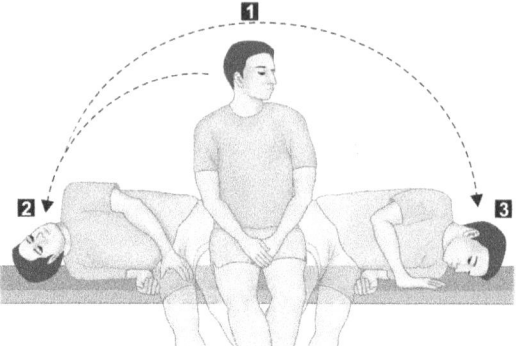

Fig. 32.14: Demonstrating Semont maneuver.

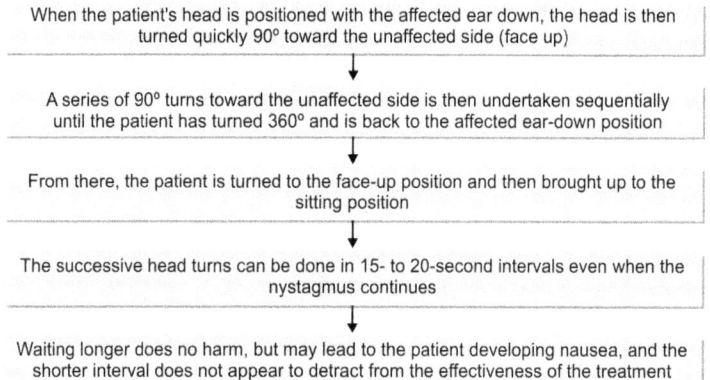

Fig. 32.15: Sequence of Lempert 360-(Barbeque) degree roll maneuver.

unilateral vestibular lesion. Initially, the exercises performed are slow gradually increasing speed as patient tolerates the movement. The patient should experience an increase in symptoms with movement. The exercises performed should be for at least 1 minute several times each day for adaptation to occur. The head is moved at varying frequencies in both horizontal and vertical planes. The advantage of these exercises is that they are low-cost and effective.

Gaze Stability Exercises

A card or a target with words on it (foveal target) is taped in front of the patient so that the patient can read it. The patient first moves his

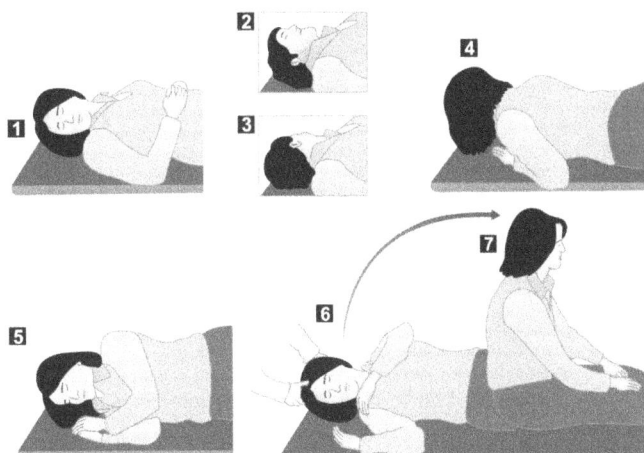
Fig. 32.16: Lempert 360-(Barbeque) degree roll maneuver.

head horizontally and then vertically for 1 minute keeping the words in focus.

Repeat the above exercise with a large pattern or without any background and gradually progress to a card with challenging background (Figs. 32.17A to C).
- In the chronic stage, the patient fixates on a visual target placed on the wall in front while gently bounces up and down on a trampoline (otoliths stimulation).
- Patients should be cautioned that the exercises may make them dizzy or nauseated but that they should try to continue for full 1 to 2 minutes, resting between the exercises.

The exercises should be performed three times a day and gradually increased to five times a day.

Postural, Balance and Gait Stability Exercises
- Patient stands with feet as close together as possible with one or both hands touching the wall to maintain balance if needed. Turn the head to the right and to the left for 1 minute without stopping. Repeat the exercise with feet closer together.
- Practice turning the head while walking. Initially practice near a wall to prevent falls.
- Stand with feet close together. Outstretch the hands in front then bring arms close to the body and lastly keep the arms folded

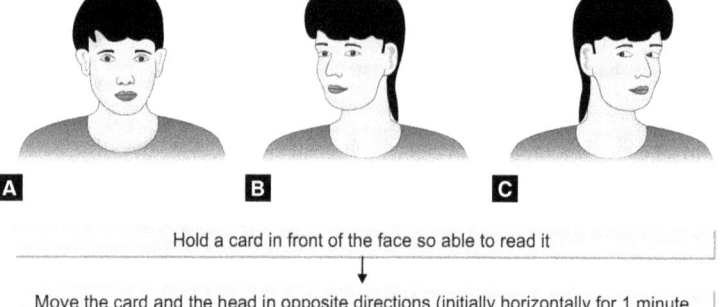

| Hold a card in front of the face so able to read it |
| ↓ |
| Move the card and the head in opposite directions (initially horizontally for 1 minute then vertically) keeping the words in focus |

Figs. 32.17A to C: Gaze stability exercises.

across the chest. Maintain each position for 15 seconds. Repeat the exercises by standing in tandem stance position, i.e. by placing one feet in front of the other.

Progression
- Repeat the above exercise with eyes closed
- In standing, shift weight from one leg to the other
- Stand on a cushioned surface (sofa cushion)
- Walk backward. The difficulty is increased by asking the patient to count backward while walking
- Walk in a large circle then walk in smaller circles and finally in figure of eight
- Walk on ramps and uneven surface
- Balance training on dynamic surface like vestibular ball or a trampoline
- In the community, walk in a mall when it is least crowded. Practice walking in the same direction as the flow of traffic or against the flow of traffic.

Desensitizing and Conditioning Exercises Program

Patients with vestibular dysfunction often significantly deconditioned due to inactivity and fearfulness of fall. Such patients are mostly advised to begin a regular walking program to not only prevent deconditioning but also to provide realistic balance challenges to the CNS, e.g. walking on uneven terrain, crossing a road, etc. Initially, they are advised to walk for 15–20 minutes daily gradually increasing to 30 minutes daily and later encouraged to walk in a park and shopping mall. Patients can be encouraged to return to recreational activities like golf, tennis, badminton, that will help to improve their fitness. Patients with unilateral vestibular lesion can safely perform swimming; however, they should not swim alone. Patients with bilateral vestibular loss, swimming is not advisable as under water, without visual cues, they may not know which way is up.

Machine-based Rehabilitation Techniques include Simulation-based Treatment

Machine-based rehabilitation provides feedback. Feedback speeds up the rehabilitation process through task understanding and performance accuracy maintaining patient's motivation and enhancing rehabilitation outcomes. The different equipment used in machine-based rehabilitation are as follows:

Optokinetic Drum and Disks

To facilitate rehabilitation of gaze stability at various speeds, direction and frequency of movement, motor driven optokinetic drums and disks are used for better carryover to daily function. The patient is safely secured in standing position and instructed to focus on a particular spot while the disk or drum rotates in a clockwise or counterclockwise direction at varying speeds from very slow to very fast.

Dynamic Posturography

It consists of a moving platform which trains the patients to rely on remaining vestibular input, particularly in condition with eyes closed. Training of weight shifts and stability limits is also possible.

Virtual Reality

Virtual reality technology offers complex sensory environment in the physical world in the controlled environments of the laboratory. The patients are so immersed in the environment that they feel that they are a part of the same. It is a laboratory created synthetic environment with precise control over a large number of physical variables, which improves behavior while recording physiological and kinematic responses. Patients are exposed to unpredictability of visual environment, e.g. head mounted display: Patients wear this device and can freely move while interacting with the visual images. Video capture: It permits the patients to observe themselves interacting with virtual objects in the laboratory.

Home Rehabilitation Videos

These are videos of optokinetic drum and disk. The patients can use these videos at home with progressive sessions—in different positions, clockwise and counterclockwise, at different distances, speeds and different support surfaces.

Index

Page numbers followed by f refer to figure, and t refer to table

A

Abscess, epidural 207
Academic skills 176
Achilles tendinitis 71
Activator technique 43
Active exercise 29, 30
    with passive effect 30
Active movements 12, 29
    and proprioceptive training 26
    under local anesthesia 29
Actual dysfunctional conditions, resolution of 60
Acupressure 13
Acupuncture 13
Additional tests 12
Adhesion formation, prevention of 27
Adjustive instrument 43
Agonist contraction 76, 77
A-icing 127
All on four 123f
Ampulla 202
Analgesia 3
Ankle 139
    splints/braces 147
    sprains 60
        acute 72
        chronic 72
Antagonist, teversal of 168
Anticoagulant medication 72
Apical segment
    anterior 188
    posterior 188
Aquarian age healing 43
Arm, dynamic reversal of 169f
Arnholz muscle adjusting 43
Arnold-Chiari
    malformation 207
    syndrome 53
Arrhythmia, cardiac 187
Arthritis 60
    inflammatory 20
Arthrokinematic 7
    motion 48
Articular strain, ligamentous 56
Articulatory technique 39
Articulatory treatment system 39
Artificial airway 187
Asthma 187
Atelectasis 187
Atlas orthogonality technique 43
Attention, regulation of 176
Autism spectrum disorders 177
Autogenic inhibition 78, 84

B

Back pain 72
Backing paper
    from center, tearing of 114f
    removal of 113, 113f
Ball pits 177
Ballistic stretching 76, 77
Bandy seminars 43
Barbecue role maneuver 213
Basal ganglia syndromes 213
Basal segment
    anterior 189
    posterior 190
Basic Brunnstrom movement therapy 136
Belt traction techniques 17

Bent leg raise technique 17
Bioenergetic synchronization technique 43
Biokinesiology 43
Biomagnetic technique 43
Blair upper cervical technique 43
Bleeding organ 55
Blisters 27
Blood-borne diseases 73
Bloodless surgery 43
Bobath concept 132
Body 9
  and brain, specialization of 177
  fluids, movement of 38
  integration 43
  percept 176
  position 150
  possesses self-regulatory mechanisms 38
  squeeze 178
Bone secondaries 61
Bony element, malpositioning of 83
Bony labyrinth 197, 200f
Brain
  injury 61
  UMN lesion, dysfunction of 207
Brandt Daroff exercises 213
Breathing 117
British Bobath Tutors Association 133
British School of Osteopathy 11
Bronchiectasis 187
Bronchopulmonary segments 187, 191f
Bronchospasm 192
Bruininks oseretsky test 178
Brunnstrom movement therapy 136
  evaluation 137
Brush stroke 74
Burn 192
  scars 72
Bursitis, non-acute 72

C

Cancer 72
Capsulitis 25
Cardiac failure 187
Carpal tunnel syndrome 71
Cassette tape recorder 177
Cavus foot 60
Cawthorne Cooksey exercises 215
Central nervous system 23
  neoplasms of 207
Central vestibular dysfunction 207
Cerebellar
  degenerations 213
  functions 210
  ischemia 207
Cerebral
  ischemia 207
  palsy 177
  vascular accidents 61
Cervical
  disc pathology, acute 53
  extension sustained natural apophyseal glides 17
  facet joint 27
  flexion sustained natural apophyseal glides 17
  rotation sustained natural apophyseal glides 17
  spine
    examination 210
    instability 53
Cervicocollic reflex 206
Cervico-ocular reflex 205
Cervicospinal reflex 206
Chapman's reflexes 40
Chest
  physiotherapy 186
  wall pain 192
Chiro plus kinesiology 43
Chiroenergetics 43
Chirometry 43
Chiropractic 5, 41
  adjustments, alternative 43
  concept 43
  distortion analysis 43
  manipulative reflex technique 43
  neuro-biomechanical analysis 43
  philosophy of 42
  spinal biophysics 43

Chiropractors, mixed 42
Choke system 43
Chronic joint swelling associated with sprains/strains 72
C-icing 127
Collins method 43
Combination therapy 178
Complex
  motor skills 176
  regional pain syndrome 60, 181
Compression 12, 63
  technique 18
  treatments 18
Concave convex rule 22
Concept therapy 43
Conjunction 63
Contract relax 76, 77
Contraction, concentric 140
Coordination, abnormal 134
Coping theory 179
Cranial
  handle 52
  technique 44
Craniopathy 44
Critical care units 186
Crocks principle 16
Cryotherapy 46
Cupula 202
Cyriax
  divide tissues 26
  mobilization techniques 24
    principles 24
    treatment 26
  soft tissue 69

D

D1 extension 153, 154*f*, 155*f*, 156
D1 flexion 153, 154*f*, 155, 155*f*
D2 extension 153, 154*f*, 155*f*, 156, 156*f*
D2 flexion 153, 154*f*, 155*f*, 156, 156*f*
Deep friction 26, 27
  massage, effects of 27
Deep vein thrombosis 72

Degenerative
  joint conditions 60
  neutral conditions 61
  spinal conditions 60
Dequervain's syndrome 71
Derangement syndrome 34-36
  features of 35
Developmental therapy 179
Direct treatment modalities 39
Directional non-force technique 44
Disc
  herniation 61
  traction 51
Distraction technique 44
Disturbed agonist-synergist-antagonist coordination 134
Diversified technique 44
Dix-Hallpike manuever test 210, 211
  modified 210, 211
Dorsiflexion 139
Dysdiadochokinesia 210
Dysfunctional syndrome 34-36

E

Edema 109
Education council on osteopathic principles 79
Elbow 139
  joint 22
Electrodiagnostic tests 12
Embolus, pulmonary 192
Encephalitis 207
Endocrine disorders 55
Endolymphatic fluid 202
Endo-nasal technique 44
Energy 9
  engaging 40
Epicondylitis
  lateral 71
  medial 71
Eplye's maneuver 213, 215*f*
  sequence of positions of 214*f*
Ergonomics 46

Exercises
　　coordination 213
　　habituation 213
　　therapeutic 46
Explicit motor imagery 183
　　training 184
Extension
　　abduction-internal rotation
　　　　with knee
　　　　　　extension 156
　　　　　　flexion 156
　　adduction-external rotation with
　　　　knee flexion 156
　　left lateral flexion-left
　　　　rotation 157, 158
　　right lateral flexion-right
　　　　rotation 157, 158
Extensor pollicis longus 111
Exteroceptive stimulation 140
Extracellular matrix 70
Extremity technique 44
Eye-hand coordination 176

F

Facet
　　distraction 51
　　gliding 51
Facial
　　correction 107, 108
　　lower extremity 142
　　muscles, facilitation of 163
　　proprioceptive neuromuscular
　　　　facilitation 163
　　　　principles of 163
　　upper extremity 142
Facilitated positional release 40, 63
　　absolute contraindications 64
　　application 65
　　history 63
　　important points 64
　　indications 63
　　mechanism of effect 64
　　relative contraindications 63
Facilitation techniques 126, 135

Fan strip 112f
Fascia 108
　　correction taping technique
　　　　114, 115
Fasciculus, medial longitudinal 203
Fast stroke 74
Fetal alcohol syndrome 177
Fever 144
Fibromyalgia pain 60
Fibrosis, cystic 187
Finger to nose rule out
　　dysmetria 210
Flexed posture 122
Flexion 57
　　abduction-internal rotation
　　　　with knee
　　　　　　extension 156
　　　　　　flexion 156
　　adduction-external rotation
　　　　with knee
　　　　　　extension 155
　　　　　　flexion 155
　　lateral flexion-rotation 157
　　left lateral flexion-left
　　　　rotation 157
　　right lateral flexion-right
　　　　rotation 157
Forearm 139
　　support 123, 123f
Fossa, posterior 207
Four taping techniques 114
Fracture 61, 72, 192
　　non-union 75
　　recent 20
　　unhealed 75
　　unstable 64
Freeman chiropractic procedure 44
Frontalis muscle 163
　　facilitation of 164f
Functional articular rolling 48, 49
Fundamental chiropractic 44

G

Gait
　　activity 178

dysfunction 177
exercises 213
Gaze stability exercises 216, 218*f*
Gentamicin ototoxicity 213
Glenohumeral joint
    co-contraction 123
Global energetic matrix 44
Global listening 55
Gluteus maximus 6
Golgi tendon organ 81, 130
Gonstead technique 44
Gross motor development,
    sequence of 122
Gua Sha technique 68

H

Hair cells 201
Hamstring muscles 6
Handlebar 68*f*
Hard end feel 75
Head
    injury associated imbalance 213
    thrust test 210
Headache 60
    cervicogenic 17
    sustained natural apophyseal
        glides 17
Heart disease 144
Heat therapy 46
Heavy loads, carrying 178
Heel pain 71
Hematoma 27, 72, 75
Hemiplegia 134
Hemoptysis, sever 187
Herring cervical technique 44
High velocity
    low amplitude 39
    thrust technique 3
Hip 139
    joint 22
    pain 72
Hold relax 76, 77, 171
Holographic diagnosis and
    treatment 44

Homeostasis 42
Homolateral limb synkineses 138
Horizontal semicircular canal 198,
    212*f*
Howard system 44
Hydraulic technique 52
Hydrocephalus 207
Hyper-extend lumbar spine 36
Hyper-retract head and neck 36
Hypersensitivity 72
Hypertension
    sever 187
    uncontrolled 72
Hypertonia 125
Hypertonicity 125
Hypomobility 19
Hypoperfusion 207
Hypotension, sever 187
Hypotonia 125

I

I strip 111*f*
Infection 72, 75, 83
Infraspinatus tendinitis 29
Inhibition techniques 129, 135
Injection and infiltration technique
    27, 32
Instrument assisted soft tissue
    mobilization 67
    contraindications 72
    history 67
    indications 71
    techniques 73
Intermittent manual traction 13
International Bobath Instructors
    Training Association 133
International Seminar of Ortho-
    paedic Manipulative Therapy 11
Intervertebral disc prolapse 35
Isometric contraction 84, 140
Isotonic
    concentric contraction 84
    eccentric contraction 84

J

Joint 2, 30, 35, 57
  concept 50
  displacement 3
  distraction 129
  examination and treatment, Kaltenborn method of 11
  gaping 48
  history 50
  homeostatic kinetics of 48
  hypermobility of 75
  manipulation 78
  manual mobilization of 11
  mechanics 109
  metacarpal 27
  mobilization 13, 74, 76, 78
  movement 75
    loss of 8
  pain 48
  play 20
  position
    in mobilization techniques 20
  sense 137
  range of motion 149
  squeeze 178
  support 107, 108
  techniques 51
Jones technique 61

K

Kaltenborn method 11
Kaltenborn-Evjenth orthopedic manual therapy 10, 11
Keck method of analysis 44
Kidney infections 72
Kinesiological tape 104, 105f, 106-108, 109t
  acrylic glue pattern 106f
  application for shoulder impingement syndrome 104f
  clinical comparisons 109
  effects of 106
  properties of 105
  strips 110

Kinesiology 43
  clinical 43
King Tetrahedron concept 44
Knee 108, 139
  joint 22
Krishna's kinetikinetic manual therapy 8, 47
  contraindications 48
  indications 48
  joint mobilization techniques 47
  principles 47
  techniques 48

L

Labyrinth, membranous 199
Labyrinthine 204
Lateral medullary syndrome 207
Learning disability 177
Left right discrimination training 183
Leg raise techniques 17
Lemond brainstem technique 44
Lempert 360-degree roll maneuver 215, 217f
  sequence of 216f
Lesion, exact location of 27
Levator palpebrae superioris 163
  facilitation of 164f
Ligament 28, 57
  sprains 72
  technique 114
Light touch 126
Limb synergies 137, 139
Lingula 189
Lingular segment
  inferior 189
  superior 189
Logan basic technique 44
Low-amplitude spinal manipulation 43
Lower limb
  extensor synergy of 139
  manual muscle testing 210
  patterns of 155

Lumbar
 discogenic technique 64
 lordosis, exaggerated 6
 spine 17
  segments 6
Lumbrical grip 151*f*
Lung
 contusion 192
 segments 187
Lymphatic correction taping technique 14, 115
Lymphatic drainage 107, 109

M

M2T blade 68*f*
Machine-based rehabilitation techniques 219
Macula 201
Maitland's mobilization 19
Malignancy 20, 207
Manipulation 3, 4, 13, 19, 30
 medicine-assisted 44
 techniques 27, 30
Manipulative physiotherapy, Maitland concept of 19
Manual therapy 1
 effects of 3
 history 1
 types of 2
Masseter temporalis muscle 166
Master energy dynamics 44
Matos maneuver 52, 53*f*
Mawhiney scoliosis technique 44
Mckenzie method 7, 8
 of mechanical diagnosis and therapy 33
  classification 34
  concept 34
  evaluation 34
Mctimody technique 44
Mears technique 44
Mechanical ventilation 187
Mechanoceptors, stimulation of 51
Medical training therapy 14

Meniere's syndrome 213
Meningitis 207
Mentalis
 facilitation of 166*f*
 muscle 165
Meric technique system 44
Metacapophalangeal joint 151
Microarticulatory oscillation, types of 66
Micromanipulation 44
Mind 9
Mirror therapy 182*f*, 184
 training 185
Mobilization 2, 3, 19
 effects of 22
 grades of 21
 with movement 17
  concept of 15
Modulation disorders 177
Motility 55
Motion
 intolerance, idiopathic 213
 palpation 44
 sickness 207
Motor
 assessment battery for children 178
 control during movements 149
 control issues 71
 co-ordination 149
 disturbance, components of 134
 functions 210
 output 204
 planning 176
 proficiency, Bruininks oseretsky test 178
 recovery, stages of 137, 138
 relearning program 145, 146
Movement
 directional preference of 34
 disturbed direction of 150
Mulligan belt 17
Mulligan concept 15
Multifactorial disequilibrium 213

Multiple sclerosis 61, 207
Muscle 3, 25, 29, 35, 57
   Contraction
      disturbed sequence of 134
      disturbed timing of 134
   contracture 83
   control 118
   edematous 60
   elongation 75
   energy technique 3, 4, 39, 76, 78, 79, 81
      application 83
      father of 80
      guideline 84
      history 79
      techniques 84
   fatigue 149, 150
   function 107
   infrahyoid 167
   normalize hypertonic 65
   palpation 44
   recruitment issues 71
   response testing 44
   shortening 75
   soreness, postexercise 75
   spasm 19, 109
   spasticity 63
   spindle gamma loop 65f
   strains 72
   strength 118
      and endurance 149
   stretching of 75
   taping technique 114
   tears 27
   tone 81, 125
      normal 133
   weakness 83, 109
Muscular
   facilitation 3
   inhibition 3
   reflexogenic effects 3
Musculoskeletal
   deformity 210
   disorders 32
   dysfunctions 60
   function 210
   and reduce pain 79
   imbalances 72
   injuries 75, 118
   pain, diseases causing 83
   synchronization and stabilization technique 44
Myocardial infarction, recent 187
Myofascia, stretching of 76
Myofascial pain and restrictions 71
Myofascial release 3, 4, 76, 78
   indirect 40
Myositis ossificans 72

N

Natural apophyseal glides 8, 16
Neck
   pain 71
   patterns of 157
   proprioceptive neuromuscular facilitation patterns of 157f
Neonatal respiratory distress syndrome 187
Neoplastic disorders 72
Nerve 25
   release 40
   root compression, sever 20
   signal interference 44
   structures, disorder of 27
Network chiropractic 44
Neural stretching 3, 4
Neural structure 3
Neural tissue mobilization 13, 76, 78
Neurodevelopmental treatment 132
Neuro-emotional technique 44
Neurokinetic therapy 173
   technique 173
   theoratical basis 173
Neuro-lymphatic reflex technique 45
Neuroma, acoustic 213
Neuromotor performance, clinical observation of 178
Neuro-musculoskeletal system, mechanical disorders of 41

Neuro-organizational technique 44
Neurotransmitter disease 177
Neurovascular reflex technique 45
Nimmo receptor-tonus technique 45
Non-progressive neurological
    disorders 213
Nordic system 11
Normal stress-short tissues 35
Normal tissues-bad stress 35
Normal vestibular system
    anatomy of 196
    physiology of 196
Norwegian system 11
Nucleus, medial vestibular 203
Nystagmus 210, 211

O

Occipital
    lower extremity 142
    upper extremity 142
Oculocervical reflex 78, 82
Oleshy 21st century technique 45
Open wound 72, 192
Optokinetic drum and disks 219
Orbicularis oculi 163
    facilitation of 164f
Orbicularis oris
    facilitation of 165f
    muscle 165
Organ
    infected 55
    inflamed 55
Oro-facial function 146
Orthopedic manual therapy
    research 14
Ortman technique 45
Oscillation 3, 4, 13
Osteogenesis imperfecta 144
Osteomyelitis 72
Osteopathic
    manipulative
        procedures, treatment
            manual of 80
        treatment 39
    philosophy, basic principles of 38

principles 37
treatment, techniques of 39
Osteopathy 5, 37
Osteoporosis 20, 53, 60, 61, 72, 83, 144
Osteoporotic bone 192
Otoconia 201
Otolithic membrane 200
Otolithic organs 201f
Overall rehabilitation program,
    part of 181f

P

Pain 19, 109, 149
    abdominal 60
    acute 75
    alleviating 60
    cervicothoracic 60
    during motion 71
    gate mechanism 3
    idiopathic 20
    inhibition 3
    intermittent 35
    perception 51
    post-surgical 60
    post-traumatic 60
    postural 150
    psychological 20
    reduction 23
    release phenomenon 18
    relief 27, 107, 108
        joint mobilization 13
Painless
    adjusting, Collins method 43
    chiropractic, Buxton technical
        course of 43
Palpate appropriate tender point 62
Palpation 12
Pancreatitis 60
Parallel bars and canes 147
Parkinson's disease 207
Passive movements 3, 12, 26
Passive soft tissue
    mobilization 13
    movements 12

Patellar tendinitis 71
Peak expiratory flow rate 193
Pelvis
    patterns of 160
    proprioceptive neuromuscular
        facilitation patterns
        of 160f, 161f
Perceptual motor
    foundations 176
    skills 176
Performance, abnormal
    functional 134
Performing functional movement
    patterns, ability of 135
Perianal posture reflex technique 45
Peri-articular tissues, stretching
    of 51, 76
Perilymphatic
    fistula 213
    fluid 202
Peripheral nerve, stretching of 76
Peripheral sensory apparatus,
    components of 196
Peripheral vestibular
    apparatus 197
    dysfunction 207
Pettibon spinal biomechanics
    technique 45
Phasic movement pattern 122
Phobic postural vertigo 213
Physiology 81
Pierce-Stillwagon technique 45
Pilates 116
    benefits of 118
    principles 116
Pillow crashing 178
Pinch grip 29
Pivot pattern 122, 122f
Placebo 3
Plantar
    fasciitis 71
    flexion 140
        inversion 140
Pneumothorax 187

Polarity technique 45
Positional release therapy 57
Postural control, loss of 134
Postural correction 36, 46
Postural drainage 186
    contraindications 187
    goals of 186
    indications 187
    limitations of 194
Postural syndrome 34-36
Posture
    greater awareness of 118
    imbalance patterns 45
Posturography, dynamic 219
Pregnancy 20, 72
Procerus muscle 164
Progression 147
Proprioceptive neuromuscular
    facilitation 148, 149
    stretching 76, 77
Proprioceptive stimulation
    exercises 213
Psoriasis 27
Punctures 12
Pure chiropractic technique 45

Q

Quick stretch 128

R

Raimiste's phenomenon 138
Ramps 177
Range of motion 3, 4, 48, 69,
    109, 171, 210
    loss of 35
    pain free full 35
Reaver's 5th cervical key 45
Receptor tonus technique 45
Reciprocal inhibition 78, 82, 84
Reflex
    creeping 142
        effects of 143
        sequence 143f
    hierarchical theory 133

Index

locomotion 142
   principle of 142
   rolling 142, 143
   sympathetic dystrophy 72
Relaxation 149
   joint mobilization 13
   post-isometric 81
   techniques 46
Releasing trapped intra-articular meniscoids 51
Respiratory
   conditions 55, 60
   problems 53
Resting muscle tone 51
Reverse headache sustained natural apophyseal glides 17
Rheumatoid
   arthritis 72
   disorders 27
Rhomberg test 210
Rhythmic
   rotation 135
   stabilization 170
Riddler reflex technique 45
Risorius and zygomaticus
   facilitation of 166f
   muscle 165
Roll over 122f
Rood's approach 119
   muscle groups 119
Rood's basic assumption 119
Rood's treatment techniques 125
Rotator cuff tendinitis 71
Rule out vertebrobasilar insufficiency 210

S

Saccades 210
Saccule 200
Sacro-occipital technique 45
Sacrospinalis muscles 6
Sample vestibular assessment form 208f
Scan stroke 73, 74f
Scapula 139
   depression 139
   patterns of 158
   proprioceptive neuromuscular facilitation patterns of 159f, 160f
   protraction 139
   retraction 139
Scapular co-contraction 123
Scars 72
   post-surgical 71
   tissue 74
      formation 75
   traumatic 71
Selective tissue tension 25
Self-headache sustained natural apophyseal glides 17
Semicircular canal 197
   anterior 198, 210, 210t, 211f
   horizontal 211
   lateral 198
   orientation of 198f
   posterior 198, 211, 211t
Semont maneuver 215, 216f
   sequence of 215f
Sensorimotor 179
Sensory
   defensiveness 177
   evaluation 137
   integration 174
      and praxis test 178
      disorder 177
      levels of 176
      theory, postulates of 174
   integration therapy 174
      history 174
      indications 177
      materials used 177
      mechanism 175
      precautions 179
      principles 176
      sample activities 177
   interaction with balance, clinical test of 178

motor integration, combined test for 210
possessing
    evaluation of 178
    disorder 177
    profile 178
    system, primary 176
Shin splints 72
Shoulder 139
    joint 22
    rhythmic stabilization of 170f
Skin lesions 55
Slow stroke 74, 129
Smooth pursuit 210
Soft tissue
    adhesions 75
    mobilization 13
        active facilitated 13
    orthopedics 45
    techniques 39
    stretching of 76
    manipulation 3, 4, 76, 78
Sole sensation 137
Somatic dysfunction
    absence of 64
    acute 63
    alleviation of 56
    chronic 63
Somatosensory reflexes 206
Somatosynthesis 45
Soreness, post-treatment 62
Souques' phenomenon 138
Southern California sensory integration tests 178
Space taping techniques 114
Spasticity 83, 134
Spears painless system 45
Speech disturbances 177
Speed test 137, 139
Spinal
    biomechanical engineering 43
    injury 61
    manipulation, types of 31
    mobilization with
        arm movements 17
        leg movements 17

stress 45
touch technique 45
Spine
    stabilization of 118
    unstable 20
Spondylolisthesis 20
Spondylotherapy 45
Squeeze technique 18
Static stretching, active 76
Stenosis, vertebral 20
Steroids, long-term use of 20
Stiffness 19, 22
Still technique 40, 66
Stimulus reflex effector technique 45
Straight chiropractors 42
Straight leg raise with
    compression 17
    traction 17
Strain counterstrain 57
    advantages 58
    application 60
    guidelines 62
    history 57
    physiology 59
Stress fracture 83
Stressology 45
Stretch 152
    joint mobilization 13
Stretching
    active 76
    dynamic 76
    passive 76
    techniques 75
        application 75
    types of 75
Strips, types of 110
Stroke 61, 207
    types of 73
Superior canal dehiscence syndrome 207
Supine withdrawal 122f
Suprahyoid muscle 167
Surgery 192
    recent 55

Sweep stroke 74
Swiss ball 177
　activity 178
Symmetrical symptoms, central of 36
Synovitis 25, 72
Syphilis 207

T

Tactile
　activities 177
　sense 176
　stimulation 140
Temporomandibular joint 27
Tendon 28, 35
　pressure 131
Tension
　balanced ligamentous 39
　balanced membranous 40
Thermal
　evaluation 56
　stimulation 127
Thermo-hydro-electro therapy 13
Thompson terminal point
　technique 45
Thorax, skin infections of 192
Thrombophlebitis 72
Thrust 3, 31
　technique 21
Thumb performs friction 29
Tibialis posterior tendinitis 71
Tieszen technique 45
Tissue
　acute injury of 75
　adhesion, breaking of 51
　characteristics 12
　contractile 25
　integrity, compromised 72
　resistance, types of 30
To-and-fro movements 28
Toes 139, 140
Toftness technique 45
Tone
　abnormal 134
　normalization of 125
Tonic labyrinthine reflex 138

Tonic lumbar reflex 138
Tonic neck reflex 204, 206
　asymmetric 137
　symmetric 138
Tonic reflexes 137
Tonic thumb reflex 138
Top notch viseral techniques 45
Torsion 63
Torticollis 45, 60
Touch sensation 137
Toxins 207
Traction 12, 31
　techniques 17
Translatoric joint play movements 12
Translatoric spinal manipulation 50
Transverse friction 28
Trapezium, capsules of 27
Trauma 192, 207
Trigger finger 72
Trigger point therapy 46
Trunk
　heavy work of 122
　patterns of 157
　proprioceptive neuromuscular
　　facilitation patterns of 158f
Truscott technique 45
Tuberculosis, pulmonary 192
Tumor 72, 83, 192
Tunnel walk 178
Two leg rotation technique 17

U

Ulcer 27
Ungerank specific low force
　chiropractic technique 45
Union fracture, delayed 75
Unstable angina 187, 192
Upper and lower extremities, flexion
　of 122
Upper cervical
　spine, injuries of 53
　technique 45
　traction 17
Upper limb
　flexor synergy of 139

function 146
patterns of 153
Upper lobe 188
Utricle 200
Utricular macula 201

V

Vaccination, recent 144
Variable force technique 45
Varicose veins 72
Verbal commands 135, 151
Vertebrobasilar syndrome 53
Vertigo 213
    adaptation exercises 213
    benign paroxysmal 210
        positional 207, 213
    central 213
    migraine associated 207
    paroxysmal positional 195
    post-traumatic 213
    psychogenic 213
Vestibular activities 178
Vestibular dysfunction 207
    causes of 206
    classification of 206
    nonotogenic causes of 207t
    otogenic causes of 207t
Vestibular end organ 204
Vestibular input, central processing of 203
Vestibular neuritis 45
Vestibular neuronitis 207
Vestibular nucleus 203, 203f
    inferior 203
    lateral 203
    location of 197f
    superior 203
Vestibular rehabilitation 195
    history 195
    therapy 195
        indications of 213, 213t
        principles of 212, 212f
        program 213, 213t
Vestibular sense 176

Vestibular stimuli 130, 210
Vestibular system function, mechanism of 196f
Vestibule 199
Vestibulocollic reflex 205
Vestibulo-ocular reflex 196
Vestibulopathy, bilateral 207
Vestibulospinal reflex 204
Vibration 13, 128, 192
Vibratory/stimulatory technique 56
Visceral manipulation 40, 54
    basics 54
    contraindications 55
    diagnosis 55
    indications 55
Visual and auditory senses 176
Visual input 196
Visual motor integration 176
Visual perception 176
Visualization 177
Visuo-motor functions 210
Vitamin deficiency 207
Vojta therapy 141, 142
    contraindications 144
    fundamentals of 142
    history 141
    indications 143
    principles of 142
Von Fox combination technique 45
VOR reflex stimulation exercises 213
VSR stimulation exercises 213

W

Wallenberg's syndrome 207
Western cerebral palsy centre 133

X

X strip 112f

Y

Y strip 112f

Z

Zindler reflex technique 45

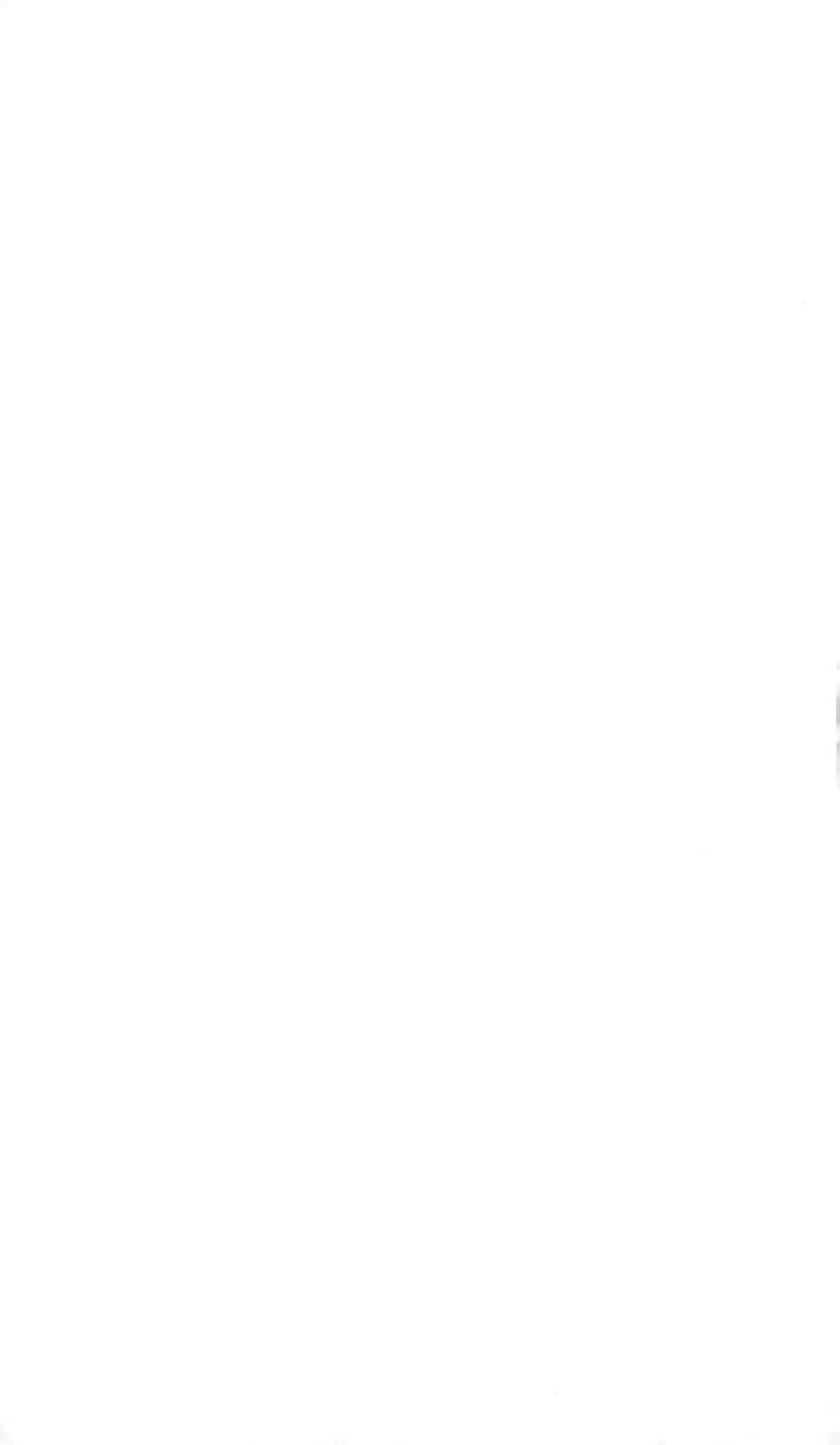

EU GSPR Authorised Reprsentative
Logos Europe, 9 rue Nicolas Poussin
1700, La Rochelle, France
Phone: +33 (0) 6 67 93 73 78
E-mail: contact@logoseurope.eu

www.ingramcontent.com/pod-product-compliance
Ingram Content Group UK Ltd.
Pitfield, Milton Keynes, MK11 3LW, UK
UKHW021832140426
5217IPUK00021B/1396